T0234738

Energy-Efficient Algorithms and Protocols
for Wireless Body Sensor Networks

Rongrong Zhang • Jihong Yu

# Energy-Efficient Algorithms and Protocols for Wireless Body Sensor Networks

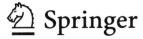 Springer

Rongrong Zhang
College of Information Engineering
Capital Normal University
Beijing, China

Jihong Yu
School of Information and Electronics
Beijing Institute of Technology
Beijing, China

ISBN 978-3-030-28582-1     ISBN 978-3-030-28580-7   (eBook)
https://doi.org/10.1007/978-3-030-28580-7

This Springer imprint is published by the registered company Springer Nature Switzerland AG.
The registered company address is: Gewerbestrasse 11, 6330 Cham, Switzerland

# Preface

Wireless Body Sensor Networks (WBSNs), which are designed and developed for human body to monitor, manage, and transmit the real-time physiological parameters, have been experiencing ever-increasing deployment in a variety of promising applications, such as medical monitoring, sport activities monitoring, and consumer electronics. On account of the scarce battery capability and real-time requirement in WBSNs, the fundamental problems are to prolong the network lifetime and reduce the transmission delay in WBSNs. These problems are simple to state and intuitively understandable, while of both fundamental and practical importance, and require nontrivial efforts to solve. Therefore, in this book, we present a systematic research on a number of research problems related to energy efficiency and time consumption. Specifically, we address the following problems ranging from theoretical modeling and analysis to practical algorithm design and optimization.

- Energy-efficient and reliable leader election mechanisms for WBSNs
- MAC protocol for duty-cycling WBSNs with concurrent traffic
- Multi-channel broadcast algorithms in duty-cycling WBSNs
- Energy-efficient and reliable sleep scheduling algorithms in WBSNs

In the book, we adopt a research and exposition line from theoretical modeling and analysis to practical algorithm design and optimization.

In order to reduce energy consumption to prolong the network lifetime while guaranteeing the network reliability, we start by investigating clustering-based leader election mechanisms in Chap. 2. Technically, we partition a WBSN into regions to manage sensor nodes and build the energy consumption model. Specifically, we construct a utility function with the consideration of both the residual energy and the location of the node, based on which we introduce an energy-efficient distributed leader election (EELE) algorithm. To improve energy efficiency, a distance-aware hybrid communication mode is further proposed such that a node can choose either direct communication or cooperative communication to alleviate the burden of the leader or the far node. Furthermore, we study both the reliability and total energy consumption of a region. Specifically, we develop a reliable and energy-efficient leader election (REELE) algorithm which jointly considers the reliability and residual energy of a node. The extensive simulation results demonstrate the effectiveness and the efficiency of EELE and REELE in terms of longer network lifetime, better energy characteristics, and higher throughput as well as higher reliability.

To lay the theoretical foundations for the design and optimization of MAC protocol, we then come up with a novel two-phase receiver-initiated MAC protocol for concurrent traffic based on asynchronous duty cycling for WBSNs, called C-MAC, in Chap. 3. Different from existing work in the literature, we focus on dealing with the bursty or concurrent traffic in medical applications of WBSNs, especially for intensive care patients. Specifically, C-MAC in the first phase employs the Carrier Sense Multiple Access with Collision Avoidance (CSMA/CA) of IEEE 802.15.6 standard and designs an ordering-based communication algorithm to effectively avoid collision. Moreover, C-MAC enables sensor nodes to switch to Standby Mode (SBM) to avoid idle listening and overhearing in the second phase. Theoretically, we mathematically characterize the performance of C-MAC in terms of the random delay and energy consumption by deriving the closed-form conditions on the design parameters. Finally, we conduct the extensive numerical analysis and simulation to demonstrate the correctness of theoretical results and the better effectiveness and efficiency of C-MAC than that of RI-MAC and A-MAC in terms of transmission delay and energy consumption.

As multi-channel communication can alleviate bandwidth limitations and improve the network throughput and reliability, we proceed to addressing the multi-channel broadcast problem, one of the most important tasks for network configuration in WBSNs in Chap. 4. We establish a generic broadcast problem arising in multi-channel duty-cycling WBSNs, where the sink needs to broadcast control information to all sensor nodes. Specifically, our objective is to design reliable multi-channel wake-up schedules with minimum worst-case broadcast delay while guaranteeing the full broadcast diversity regardless of clock drifts and asymmetric duty cycles and channel perceptions. To this end, we first derive the lower bound of worst-case broadcast delay with full diversity of any multi-channel broadcast algorithm and then design a suit of two multi-channel broadcast (MCB) algorithms with the latter reducing the worst-case broadcast delay of the former by up to half and further prove that our algorithms achieve guaranteed broadcast delivery within order-minimal worst-case delay in the asynchronous and heterogeneous environment both theoretically and experimentally.

We further proceed to addressing the energy-efficient and reliable sleep scheduling problem in WBSNs in Chap. 5. Different to the existing works in this field, we focus on scheduling the sensor nodes by constructing Minimum Weighted $m$-fold Dominating Set (MWmDS) where $m$ is the number of links from a node outside DS to those in DS. The key idea is to activate partial nodes at each frame to form a DS which can guarantee the network reliability such that the other nodes can fall asleep to save energy. More specifically, we first formulate the sleep scheduling in a WBSN as a problem of constructing MWmDS which is proven NP-hard. Then, we design an $H(m + \delta)$-approximation algorithm, named GAA, which globally select an optimal node that contributes to the maximum increment of a polymatroid function and residual energy to be the final dominator in each iteration. Subsequently, a simplified algorithm, named LAA, is proposed to reduce the computational complexity and execution time of GAA. In LAA, multiple dominators are elected among one-hop neighbors in each iteration. Moreover, we theoretically prove the correctness and approximation rate of our proposed algorithms. We also conduct extensive simulations, and the results confirm the efficiency of our algorithms in prolonging the network lifetime and their effectiveness in constructing an MWmDS.

Beijing, China                                                                        Rongrong Zhang
Beijing, China                                                                              Jihong Yu

# Contents

1   **Introduction** ................................................................ 1
    1.1   Overview of WBSNs.................................................... 1
    1.2   Design Requirement of WBSNs..................................... 3
    1.3   Wireless Technologies for WBSNs ................................ 4
    1.4   Open Issues and Challenges in WBSNs ............................ 6
    1.5   Book Organization .................................................... 8
    References ................................................................ 9

2   **Energy-Efficient and Reliable Leader Election Mechanisms**
    **for WBSNs** .............................................................. 11
    2.1   Introduction ........................................................... 11
        2.1.1   Context and Motivation........................................ 11
        2.1.2   Summary of Contributions ................................... 12
    2.2   Related Work .......................................................... 13
    2.3   Network Model........................................................ 15
    2.4   Proposed Energy-Efficient Leader Election Mechanism ............. 17
        2.4.1   Energy Consumption-Based Hybrid Communication
              Strategy............................................................ 17
        2.4.2   Leader Election Algorithm ................................... 18
        2.4.3   Energy-Efficient Leader Election Mechanism................. 20
        2.4.4   Performance Evaluation ....................................... 21
    2.5   Proposed Reliable and Energy-Efficient Leader Election Mechanism   28
        2.5.1   Reliability Model .............................................. 28
        2.5.2   Reliable and Energy-Efficient Communication Strategy ..... 29
        2.5.3   Total Energy Consumption Model ........................... 30
        2.5.4   Reliable Leader Election Algorithm ......................... 31
        2.5.5   Performance Evaluation ....................................... 33
    2.6   Conclusion ............................................................ 37
    References ................................................................ 38

**3   MAC Protocol for Duty-Cycling WBSNs with Concurrent Traffic**.....   39
    3.1   Introduction ...............................................................   39
          3.1.1   Context and Motivation..........................................   39
          3.1.2   Summary of Contributions ......................................   40
    3.2   Related Work ...............................................................   41
    3.3   System Model ..............................................................   43
    3.4   Overview of IEEE 802.15.6 CSMA/CA Protocol ....................   45
    3.5   C-MAC Description.........................................................   46
          3.5.1   Overview of C-MAC ............................................   46
          3.5.2   Ordering-Based Communication Algorithm ..................   47
    3.6   Delay Analysis ..............................................................   49
          3.6.1   Modeling of $T_1$.................................................   51
          3.6.2   Modeling of $T_w$ ...............................................   53
          3.6.3   Modeling of $T_o$ and $T_c$....................................   59
          3.6.4   Accuracy Evaluation.............................................   60
    3.7   Energy Consumption Analysis ...........................................   62
          3.7.1   Modeling of Energy Consumption ............................   62
          3.7.2   Accuracy Evaluation.............................................   64
    3.8   Performance Evaluation ...................................................   65
          3.8.1   Simulation Settings ..............................................   65
          3.8.2   Simulation Results and Analysis..............................   65
    3.9   Conclusion ..................................................................   69
    References ..........................................................................   70

**4   Multi-Channel Broadcast Algorithms in Duty-Cycling WBSNs**........   73
    4.1   Introduction ...............................................................   73
          4.1.1   Context and Motivation..........................................   73
          4.1.2   Summary of Contributions ......................................   75
    4.2   Related Work ...............................................................   75
    4.3   Problem Formulation ......................................................   78
          4.3.1   System Model.....................................................   78
          4.3.2   Performance Metrics.............................................   80
          4.3.3   Optimal Problem.................................................   80
    4.4   Multi-Channel Broadcast Delay Bound.................................   81
    4.5   MCB: Single-Channel Case ..............................................   83
          4.5.1   Technical Background ...........................................   83
          4.5.2   Algorithm Design................................................   84
          4.5.3   Duty Cycle Granularity..........................................   85
          4.5.4   Broadcast Delay .................................................   86
    4.6   MCB: Multi-Channel Case ...............................................   86
          4.6.1   Motivation and Algorithm Design ............................   86
          4.6.2   Broadcast Delay .................................................   88
    4.7   An Improved MCB..........................................................   88
          4.7.1   An Improved Algorithm.........................................   89
          4.7.2   Robustness Against Asymmetrical Channel Perception ......   90

4.8    Performance Evaluation .............................................. 92
       4.8.1   Performance Comparison: Reliability ........................ 92
       4.8.2   Performance Comparison: Broadcast Delay.................. 93
4.9    Conclusion .......................................................... 99
References ................................................................. 99

5   Energy-Efficient and Reliable Sleep Scheduling Algorithms
    in WBSNs ............................................................... 101
    5.1    Introduction ...................................................... 101
           5.1.1   Context and Motivation...................................... 101
           5.1.2   Summary of Contributions .................................. 102
    5.2    Related Work ..................................................... 103
    5.3    Preliminary ...................................................... 104
    5.4    System Model and Problem Statement ............................. 106
           5.4.1   System Model............................................... 106
           5.4.2   Problem Formulation ........................................ 107
    5.5    GAA: Global Approximation Algorithm ........................... 108
           5.5.1   Algorithm Design........................................... 109
           5.5.2   Algorithm Analysis ......................................... 110
    5.6    LAA: Local Approximation Algorithm............................. 111
           5.6.1   Algorithm Design........................................... 111
           5.6.2   Algorithm Analysis ......................................... 113
    5.7    Performance Evaluation .......................................... 115
           5.7.1   Simulation Settings and Performance Metrics .............. 115
           5.7.2   Simulation Results ......................................... 116
    5.8    Conclusion ....................................................... 120
    References ............................................................. 120

6   Conclusion and Perspective ............................................ 123
    6.1    Book Summary.................................................... 123
    6.2    Open Questions and Future Work ................................ 125
           6.2.1   Efficient Multicasting Algorithm ........................... 125
           6.2.2   Efficient Transmission Strategy with Energy Harvesting ..... 125
           6.2.3   Extension to Cloud Computing .............................. 126
    References ............................................................. 126

Index ....................................................................... 129

# Chapter 1
# Introduction

## 1.1 Overview of WBSNs

A wireless body sensor network (WBSN) typically consists of a collection of low-power, miniaturized, and lightweight devices with wireless communication capabilities that operate in the proximity of a human body. Generally speaking, these devices can be distinguished as three types: sensors, actuators, and personal digital assistant (PDA) [1]. The sensors can be implanted in, on, or around the human body to monitor, manage, and transmit the real-time physiological parameters such as the heartbeat, body temperature, blood pressure, electrocardiogram (ECG), and electroencephalogram (EEG). The actuators on the other hand act as drug-delivery systems equipped with a built-in reservoir to deliver the medicine on predetermined moment, triggered by an external source or immediately when sensors notice a problem. The PDA acts as a sink to collect all the information attained by the sensors and transmit it to the users (patient, nurse, physician, etc.) via an external gateway [2].

As WBSNs can provide interconnection among various devices in or around human body, it can support a large number of potential applications in several areas. The main applications can be roughly categorized into medical and non-medical applications, such as healthcare, sports and entertainment, and military and defense, etc. [3].

- *Healthcare:* This is the most promising WBSN application at a first glance. Using WBSNs in medical applications, the sensor nodes can continuously monitor the vital signals, as well as provide real-time feedback and information [4]. More specifically, the sensor nodes monitor and transmit one's physiological attributes such as blood pressure, heartbeat, and body temperature. In cases where abnormal conditions are detected, the information can be delivered and effectively processed to obtain reliable and accurate physiological estimations and allow scientists, physicians, or other medical professionals to have real-

© Springer Nature Switzerland AG 2020

R. Zhang and J. Yu, *Energy-Efficient Algorithms and Protocols for Wireless Body Sensor Networks*, https://doi.org/10.1007/978-3-030-28580-7_1

time opinions for medical diagnosis and prescription. Therefore, WBSNs can provide interfaces for diagnostics, for remote monitoring of human physiological data, for administration of drugs in hospitals and an aid to rehabilitation. In the future, it will be possible to monitor patients continuously and give the necessary medication whether they are at home, in a hospital, or elsewhere. Patients will no longer need to be connected to large machines in order to be monitored. Moreover, WBSNs cannot only detect fatal events and anomalies, they can also improve the life style of hearing and visually impaired people by methods of hearing aid, cochlear implant and artificial retina, respectively. Recent research has shown the effective realization of human emotions via speech and visual data analysis. Specifically, wearable sensing technologies have enabled emotion detection by the introduction of physical appearances throughout the body that leads to the production of signals to be measured by simple bio-sensors. For instance, fear increases respiration rate and heartbeat, which results in palm sweating and more. Therefore, one's emotional status can be monitored anywhere and anytime by monitoring emotion-related physiological signals.

- *Sport and entertainment:* In the sporting area, it will be possible to take many different readings from an athlete without having them on a treadmill in a laboratory. WBSNs can provide monitoring parameters, motion capture, and rehabilitation during the athlete's real life competition, thus the training schedules can easily be tuned based on their strengths and weaknesses. Moreover, the real-time feedback of WBSNs allows the users to prevent injuries caused by incorrect training and to plan future training to improve their performance.

  The entertainment applications consist of gaming applications and social networking. Appliances such as microphones, MP3-players, cameras, head-mounted displays, and advanced computer appliances can be used as devices integrated in WBSNs. They can be used in virtual reality and gaming purposes (game control with hand gesture, mobile body motion game, and virtual world game), personal item tracking, exchanging digital profile/business card, and consumer electronics.

- *Military and defense:* The activity of soldiers in the battlefield can be monitored more closely by WBSNs, thus it will enhance the military effect at both individual and squad level. The soldier can avoid threats based on the information about the surrounding environments provided by a set of sensors. And the commander is able to better coordinate the squad actions and tasks. Moreover, the inter-WBSN authentications play an important role in order to prevent sensitive information from being caught by the enemies. Additionally, WBSNs can also be used by policeman and fire-fighters. The use of WBSNs in harsh environments can be instrumental in reducing the probability of injury while providing improved monitoring and care in case of injury.

## 1.2   Design Requirement of WBSNs

WBSNs applications show great promise in improving the user's quality of life [5] and satisfying many of elderly people by enabling them to live safely, securely, and independently. Due to the limitations in the nature of WBSNs, it provides many design requirements which can be summarized as follows:

- *Communication range:* WBSNs allow the sensors in, on, and around the same body to communicate with each other, so 2–5 m operating communication range is enough in a WBSN.
- *Network density:* With the diversification of WBSN applications, people should be able to have sensor nodes for different applications and different body area networks on them. A typical medical network based on WBSNs is stated to have 6 nodes with a scalable configuration that supports up to 256 sensor nodes, while only one sink is allowed to exist in a WBSN. And also only 2–4 WBSNs are stated to coexist on the same person per $m^2$.
- *Data rate:* The bit rate requirement varies on a very broad range depending on the application and on the type of data to be transmitted. WBSN links should support the bit rate from less than 1 Kb/s (e.g., temperature monitoring) to 10 Mb/s (e.g., video streaming). The bit rate can refer to a single link or to multiple links, when several devices transmit/receive information to/from one coordinator at the same time.
- *Low power:* All nodes in WBSNs should be capable of transmitting at 0.1 mW ($-10$ dBm) and the maximum radiated transmission power should be less than 1 mW (0 dBm). This complies with the specific absorption rate (SAR) of the Federal Communications Commission's 1.6 W/Kg in 1 g of body tissue.
- *Latency:* The goal of monitoring applications is a collection of information in the real time, so the tight delay requirement is necessary. As specified in IEEE 802.15.6 standard [6], the latency should be less than 125 ms in medical applications and less than 250 ms in non-medical applications.
- *Coexistence:* WBSNs may interact with the Internet and other existing wireless technologies like Bluetooth, ZigBee, wireless sensor networks (WSNs), wireless local area networks (WLAN), and wireless personal area network (WPAN). Thus, WBSNs should be able to operate in a heterogeneous environment where networks of different standards cooperate among each other to transmit and receive information.
- *Interference:* Since a WBSN is most likely to encounter other WBSNs where the different types of radio interference can be encountered, inter-WBSN interference is of the utmost importance. And collision from external sensors may also lead to the interference. Additionally, the unpredictable nature of postural body movement may also introduce additional interference. Therefore, interference should be mitigated as much as possible in WBSNs to satisfy the reliable wireless communication.
- *Reliability:* Nodes should be capable of reliable communication even when the person is on the move. Although it is acceptable for network capacity to be

reduced, data should not be lost due to unstable channel conditions. Reliability of WBSNs depends upon transmission delay of packets and packet loss probability. Packet transmission procedure at MAC layer and bit error rate (BER) of channel influence packet loss probability. Appropriate channel access techniques, packet retransmission schemes, packet size, and enhanced scheduling schemes at MAC layer improve reliability.

• *Scalability:* Scalability is the essential requirement for WBSNs. The number of nodes, to collect life critical and non-critical information, varies according to the patient monitoring requirements. Easily configuration of WBSNs by adding or removing sensor nodes is required to support scalability.

These requirements may differ while considering the different operational environments and characteristics of each WBSN application.

## 1.3 Wireless Technologies for WBSNs

In order to satisfy the design requirements of WBSNs, many related wireless technologies are involved in communication among sensor nodes as well as between the sink and sensor nodes.

**Bluetooth** technology [7] was designed as a short-range wireless communication standard intended to replace the cables connecting portable and/or fixed electronic devices. The main attractive characteristics of Bluetooth are robustness, low power consumption, and low cost. Thus, it is widely used to connect a variety of personally carried devices to support data and voice applications. Bluetooth devices operate in the 2.4 GHz ISM band utilizing frequency hopping among 791 MHz channels at a nominal rate of 1600 hops/s to reduce interference. The standard specifies three classes of devices with different transmission powers and corresponding coverage ranging from 1 to 100 m. The maximum data rate is 3 Mbps.

A derived option of the Bluetooth standard is the **Bluetooth low energy (BLE)** [8], which was introduced as a more suitable option for WBSNs where less power consumption is possible using low duty cycle operation. BLE was designed to wirelessly connect small devices to mobile terminals. Those devices are often too tiny to bear the power consumption as well as cost associated with a standard Bluetooth radio, but are ideal choices for the health monitoring applications. BLE supports bit rate up to 1 Mbps and operates in the 2.45 GHz ISM band, where 40 channels, each one is 2 MHz wide, are defined. Using fewer channels for pairing devices, synchronization can be done in a few milliseconds compared to Bluetooth seconds. This benefits latency-critical WBSN applications, like alarm generation and emergency response, and enhances power saving. Its nominal data rate, low latency, and low energy consumption make BLE suitable for communication between the wearable sensor nodes and the access point. Moreover, adaptive frequency hop spread spectrum allows BLE to coexist with Wi-Fi. However, interference with other devices might be an issue as the technology operates in the 2.4 GHz ISM band. And the main drawbacks of BLE are the lack of multi-hop communication and the limited scalability, in fact only star topologies are possible.

**ZigBee** [9] defined by ZigBee specification is one of the wireless network technologies which is widely used in the low power environment. ZigBee is targeted at radio frequency applications that require a low data rate, long battery life, and secure networking, thanks to its 128-bit security support to perform authentication and guarantee integrity and privacy of message. Through the sleep mode, ZigBee enabled devices are capable of being operational for several years before their batteries need to be replaced. ZigBee technology is separated into two parts. First, ZigBee alliance designates the application layers, defining the network, security, and application software layers. Second, IEEE 802.15.4 standard [10] defines the physical and medium access control layers, where access to wireless channel is through employing unslotted/slotted carrier sense multiple access with collision avoidance (CSMA/CA) mechanism for channel access and handling guaranteed time slot (GTS) allocation and management.

**IEEE 802.15.4** [10] is a short-range (up to 100 m) communication system intended to enable applications with relaxed throughput and latency requirements in wireless personal area networks (WPAN). IEEE 802.15.4 oriented to lightweight fixed or mobile devices is of low complexity, low energy consumption and low bit rate. The main field of application of this technology is the implementation of WSNs. The network topologies supported are the star, tree, and mesh.

IEEE 802.15.4 specifies a total of 27 half-duplex channels across three frequency bands, organized as follows: (1) The 868 MHz band with just a single channel with bit rate of 20 kbps; (2) The 915 MHz band, where 10 channels with a bit rate of 40 kbps are available; (3) The 2.45 GHz ISM band with 16 channels with bit rate equal to 250 kbps. Thus, one significant disadvantage of ZigBee for WBSN applications is due to interference with WLAN transmission, especially in 2.45 GHz where numerous wireless systems operate. Another disadvantage of ZigBee is related to its low data rate, which makes it inappropriate for large-scale and real-time WBSN applications. In fact, due to the low rate, it is difficult to implement in hospitals or clinics.

IEEE Task Group TG6 was established in November 2007 to realize a standard specifically designed for WBSNs, namely **IEEE 802.15.6** which is the first WBSNs standard that serves various medical and non-medical applications and supports communication inside and around the human body. The final version was released in February 2012 [6]. IEEE 802.15.6 standard uses different frequency bands for data transmission including: the narrow band (NB), which includes the 400, 800, 900 MHz and the 2.3 and 2.4 GHz bands; the ultra-wideband (UWB), which uses the 3.2 GHz; and the human body communication (HBC), which uses the frequencies within the range of 1050 MHz. This standard is a step forward in wearable sensor networks as it is designed specifically for use with a wide range of data rates, less energy consumption, low range, ample number of nodes (256) per body area network, and different node priorities according to the application requirements. The channel access is handled using CSMA/CA or slotted Aloha access procedure.

It provides flexibility in security features, since it defines three security schemes. IEEE 802.15.6 standard can reach data rates up to 10 Mbps while being extremely low power. In addition, it can consider some movements of body and can satisfy most of the WBSN applications throughput requirements by achieving a maximum of 680 Kbps. But it is not able to meet the constraints of the emerging applications which require high quality audio or video transmissions.

Recently, **SmartBAN** [11] has been defined from the European Telecommunication Standard Institute (ETSI) in 2015 with the scope to specify a low complexity MAC protocol. The goal of the SmartBAN is to define a standard for low power devices and networks to be used in short-range link supporting, e.g., healthcare, wellness, and sport related applications operating around a human body. The key features of the SmartBAN are the use of separate channels for data (DCH) and control traffic (CCH), a guarantee for very low latency emergency messaging, and increase of channel utilization and retransmission through the use of scheduled but unused time slots by secondary users. The device operates in the ISM band within 2401–2481 MHz using a bandwidth of 2 MHz and there are available 37 DCHs and 3 CCHs. However, due to the limited coverage area and the properties and functions of SmartBAN, only a single-hop star topology is considered.

## 1.4   Open Issues and Challenges in WBSNs

Although several wireless technologies have been involved to satisfy the design requirements of WBSNs and a lot of research is going on, there still exist many open issues and challenges to be addressed, such as channel model, energy efficiency, security, authentication and privacy, etc. [12, 13]:

- *PHY layer design:* Nodes in WBSNs are scattered in or on the human body, which creates multiple transmission channels between the nodes based on their location. Thus, the channel modeling plays a crucial role in the design of PHY technologies. In the past decade, many researchers have already proposed a few channel models for the physical layer [14–17]. However, experimental channel modeling for implants and wearable devices is difficult due to involvement of human subjects and healthcare facilities, both governed by regulations. And it should be noticed that none of them take the movements of the body into account, although movements can have a severe impact on the received signal strength. Furthermore, new emerging technologies such as galvanic coupling and transformation of information via the bones offer promising results and need to be investigated more thoroughly.
- *MAC layer design:* Energy efficiency is the utmost important requirement of a good MAC protocol for WBSNs. Recently, many researchers have proposed a number of MAC protocols for WBSNs [18–20]. However, high energy efficient MAC protocols specifically for WBSNs still need to be developed, which should have the capabilities to avoid energy dissipation due to collision

of packets, overhearing of nodes, and idle listening to receive probable data packets and control packet overhead of communication. Moreover, fairness at MAC layer, high bandwidth utilization, reliable communication, minimum delay, and reduced synchronization cost are other objectives for multipurpose efficient MAC protocol. And the MAC protocol should have capabilities to accommodate communication of normal, emergency, and on-demand traffic. Furthermore, specific MAC protocols need to be developed that take into account the movement of body, i.e., the mobility of the nodes, additional low power features, the use of the human physiology such as heartbeat to ensure the time synchronization, and so on.

- *Network layer design:* Energy efficiency is one of the main goals to achieve in WBSNs for mobile and ubiquitous health monitoring with critical and non-critical conditions. Current research work for energy minimization is focused at MAC layer. However, other areas such as network layer and cross layer design need to be considered for energy minimization. A promising research track is the combination of thermal routing with more energy-efficient mechanisms [21]. Other interesting open issues are mobility support embedded in the protocol, security, interoperability, and so on. In order to design a globally optimal system, we can improve energy efficiency by integrating two or more protocol layers in a cross layer design. Therefore, research work using cross layer approach will be a prominent field to minimize energy consumption.

- *Antenna design:* As nodes are going to be put on human bodies or even implanted, their size, material, shape, and physical compatibility to human tissues are crucial. Thus, antenna design for WBSN applications is also a challenging problem due to restrictions on the size, material, and shape of the antenna [22–24]. The radio frequency environment changes with the user's age, weight gain or loss, and posture changes. Only non-corrosive and biocompatible material such as platinum or titanium can be used for implants, which results in poorer performance when compared to a copper antenna. Moreover, the shape and size of an implant antenna depends on its location and organ, which further limits the freedom of the designer. At the same time, the electronic and magnetic energy absorbed by human tissues from radio frequency circuits placed in close proximity to humans should also be concerned.

- *Energy supply:* As all WBSN devices require an energy source for data collection, processing, and transmission, development of suitable power supplies becomes paramount. Most WBSN devices are powered by batteries, which may not even be replaceable in cases where the devices are implanted in the human body; thus, techniques like remote battery recharging are important. Specifically, researchers are exploring several promising techniques such as low-power listening and wake-up radios, which are intended to minimize power consumed by idle listening. Additionally, the energy harvesting methods have been studied [25] recently to prolong the lifetime of the nodes' battery. But the energy conserving problem has not been addressed effectively in detail.

- *QoS and reliability:* Proper QoS and reliability of wireless WBSN technology is an important part in the framework of risk management of medical applications. The QoS framework should be flexible so that it can be dynamically configured to suit application requirements without unduly increasing complexity or decreasing system performance. And the reliability of the network directly affects the quality of patient monitoring and in a worst-case scenario, it can be fatal when a life-threatening event has gone undetected. Thus a reliable end-to-end transmission is necessary to guarantee that the monitored data is received correctly by the health-care professionals.

* *Security and privacy:* The communication of health-related information between sensors in a WBSN and over the Internet to servers is strictly private and confidential and should be encrypted to protect the patient's privacy. The medical staff collecting the data needs to be confident that the data is not tempered with and indeed originates from that patient. And a highly secure system may prevent paramedics from accessing critical physiological information in case of an emergency, thereby endangering the life of the person. However, the conventional security and privacy mechanisms are not suitable for WBSNs due to limited processing power, memory and energy, lack of user interface, unskilled users, longevity of devices, and global roaming. Hence, novel lightweight and resource efficient methods have to be developed for WBSNs.

## 1.5  Book Organization

In this book, we adopt a research and exposition line from theoretical modeling and analysis to practical algorithm design and optimization. Figure 1.1 illustrates the structure of the book. In the remainder of this section, we provide a high-level overview of the technical contributions of our book, which are presented sequentially in Chaps. 2–5. To facilitate readers, we adopt a modularized structure to present the results such that the chapters are arranged as independent modules, each devoted to a specific topic outlined above. In particular, each chapter has

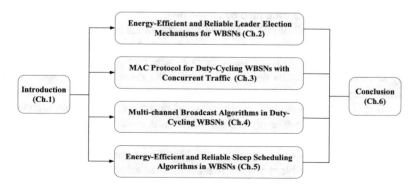

**Fig. 1.1** Book organization

its own introduction and conclusion section, elaborating the related work and the importance of the results with the specific context of that chapter. For this reason, we are not providing a detailed background or a survey of prior work here.

# References

1. R. Cavallari, F. Martelli, R. Rosini, C. Buratti, R. Verdone, A survey on wireless body area networks: technologies and design challenges. IEEE Commun. Surv. Tutorials **16**(3), 1635–1657 (2014)
2. B. Latré, B. Braem, I. Moerman, C. Blondia, P. Demeester, A survey on wireless body area networks. Wirel. Netw. **17**(1), 1–18 (2011)
3. A. Nadeem, M.A. Hussain, O. Owais, A. Salam, S. Iqbal, K. Ahsan, Application specific study, analysis and classification of body area wireless sensor network applications. Comput. Netw. **83**, 363–380 (2015)
4. M. Shu, D. Yuan, C. Zhang, Y. Wang, C. Chen, A mac protocol for medical monitoring applications of wireless body area networks. Sensors **15**(6), 12906–12931 (2015)
5. S. Movassaghi, M. Abolhasan, J. Lipman, D. Smith, A. Jamalipour, Wireless body area networks: a survey. IEEE Commun. Surv. Tutorials **16**(3), 1658–1686 (2014)
6. I.S. Association et al., IEEE standard for local and metropolitan area networks-part 15.6: wireless body area networks. IEEE Stand. Inf. Technol. **802**(6), 1–271 (2012)
7. S. Bluetooth, in *Specification of the Bluetooth System v4. 2*, Standard, Bluetooth SIG, vol. 27 (2014)
8. C. Gomez, J. Oller, J. Paradells, Overview and evaluation of Bluetooth low energy: an emerging low-power wireless technology. Sensors **12**(9), 11734–11753 (2012)
9. S. Farahani, *ZigBee Wireless Networks and Transceivers* (Newnes, Oxford, 2011)
10. D. Mirzoev et al., *Low Rate Wireless Personal Area Networks (LR-WPAN 802.15. 4 standard)* (2014). Preprint. arXiv:1404.2345
11. M. Hämäläinen, T. Paso, L. Mucchi, M. Girod-Genet, J. Farserotu, H. Tanaka, W.H. Chin, L.N. Ismail, ETSI TC SmartBAN: overview of the wireless body area network standard, in *2015 9th International Symposium on Medical Information and Communication Technology (ISMICT)* (IEEE, Piscataway, 2015), pp. 1–5
12. D.M. Barakah, M. Ammad-uddin, A survey of challenges and applications of wireless body area network (WBAN) and role of a virtual doctor server in existing architecture, in *2012 Third International Conference on Intelligent Systems Modelling and Simulation* (IEEE, Piscataway, 2012), pp. 214–219
13. Y. Du, F. Hu, L. Wang, F. Wang, Framework and challenges for wireless body area networks based on big data, in *2015 IEEE International Conference on Digital Signal Processing (DSP)* (IEEE, Piscataway, 2015), pp. 497–501
14. J. Ryckaert, P. De Doncker, R. Meys, A. de Le Hoye, S. Donnay, Channel model for wireless communication around human body. Electron. Lett. **40**(9), 1 (2004)
15. E. Reusens, W. Joseph, B. Latré, B. Braem, G. Vermeeren, E. Tanghe, L. Martens, I. Moerman, C. Blondia, Characterization of on-body communication channel and energy efficient topology design for wireless body area networks. IEEE Trans. Inf. Technol. Biomed. **13**(6), 933–945 (2009)
16. R. Chávez-Santiago, K. Sayrafian-Pour, A. Khaleghi, K. Takizawa, J. Wang, I. Balasingham, H.-B. Li, Propagation models for IEEE 802.15.6 standardization of implant communication in body area networks. IEEE Commun. Mag. **51**(8), 80–87 (2013)
17. S. van Roy, F. Quitin, L. Liu, C. Oestges, F. Horlin, J.-M. Dricot, P. De Doncker, Dynamic channel modeling for multi-sensor body area networks. IEEE Trans. Antennas Propag. **61**(4), 2200–2208 (2013)

18. S.J. Marinkovic, E.M. Popovici, C. Spagnol, S. Faul, W.P. Marnane, Energy-efficient low duty cycle MAC protocol for wireless body area networks. IEEE Trans. Inf. Technol. Biomed. **13**(6), 915–925 (2009)
19. S. Ullah, K.S. Kwak, An ultra low-power and traffic-adaptive medium access control protocol for wireless body area network. J. Med. Syst. **36**(3), 1021–1030 (2012)
20. N. Javaid, S. Hayat, M. Shakir, M. Khan, S.H. Bouk, Z. Khan, Energy efficient MAC protocols in wireless body area sensor networks-a survey (2013). Preprint. arXiv:1303.2072
21. N. Javaid, Z. Abbas, M. Fareed, Z. Khan, N. Alrajeh, M-ATTEMPT: a new energy-efficient routing protocol for wireless body area sensor networks. Procedia Comput. Sci. **19**, 224–231 (2013)
22. S.L. Cotton, W.G. Scanlon, Channel characterization for single-and multiple-antenna wearable systems used for indoor body-to-body communications. IEEE Trans. Antennas Propag. **57**(4), 980–990 (2009)
23. G.A. Conway, S.L. Cotton, W.G. Scanlon, An antennas and propagation approach to improving physical layer performance in wireless body area networks. IEEE J. Sel. Areas Commun. **27**(1), 27–36 (2009)
24. S. Ullah, H. Higgins, B. Braem, B. Latre, C. Blondia, I. Moerman, S. Saleem, Z. Rahman, K.S. Kwak, A comprehensive survey of wireless body area networks. J. Med. Syst. **36**(3), 1065–1094 (2012)
25. N. Barroca, H.M. Saraiva, P.T. Gouveia, J. Tavares, L.M. Borges, F.J. Velez, C. Loss, R. Salvado, P. Pinho, R. Gonçalves et al., Antennas and circuits for ambient RF energy harvesting in wireless body area networks, in *2013 IEEE 24th Annual International Symposium on Personal, Indoor, and Mobile Radio Communications (PIMRC)* (IEEE, Piscataway, 2013), pp. 532–537

# Chapter 2
# Energy-Efficient and Reliable Leader Election Mechanisms for WBSNs

**Chapter Roadmap** The rest of this chapter is organized as follows: Section 2.1 explains the motivation of studying leader election algorithms and summarizes the contributions. Section 2.2 gives a brief overview of related work. In Sect. 2.3, we present the network model, including the energy consumption model. Sections 2.4 and 2.5 introduce our proposed EELE and REELE algorithms in detail, respectively. Finally, we conclude the chapter in Sect. 2.6.

## 2.1  Introduction

### 2.1.1  Context and Motivation

A WBSN typically consists of a collection of low-power, miniaturized, lightweight devices with sensor capabilities on, around, or implanted in the human body. The main two types of devices can be distinguished: sensor nodes and PDA which acts as the sink. The sink is to collect all the information from sensors and transmit it to the user (patient, nurse, etc.) via an external gateway. Due to the highly extensive potential applications, WBSNs have been paid great attention in recent years.

On the account of the low power level and scare battery capacity, a fundamental problem in WBSNs is to prolong the network lifetime. Considerable researchers set out to study the relative protocols to reduce energy consumption. Thus a number of energy-efficient protocols have been conducted, among which the cluster-based mechanism extensively attracts more attention in wireless networks where the network is divided into a set of clusters with a cluster head and some normal nodes as its members.

Cluster solutions can be classified according to several criteria, such as the technique of cluster head selection and the methodology of clustering. Cluster head are responsible for collecting data from their respective members, performing some

© Springer Nature Switzerland AG 2020
R. Zhang and J. Yu, *Energy-Efficient Algorithms and Protocols for Wireless Body Sensor Networks*, https://doi.org/10.1007/978-3-030-28580-7_2

data aggregation, and forwarding the meaningful data to the base station. The data traffic loads tend to be concentrated at cluster head, which makes cluster head selection an essential step to further reducing energy consumption and extending the network lifetime.

In the past decade, numerous clustering solutions have been proposed for WSNs. While every solution deals with specific clustering challenge and/or application requirements, extending the network lifetime is the main and common objective shared by all cluster protocols. Heinzelman et al. proposed LEACH [1] that uses a probabilistic process to elect cluster head. And the task of being a cluster head is rotated between nodes to balance the energy consumption and to avoid some nodes die earlier. Besides, HEED is proposed in [2] where the cluster head is selected according to a hybrid function between node residual energy and node degree.

However, due to the typical feature of WBSNs, the existing protocols for the large-scale WSNs are not exactly applicable to the WBSNs. Therefore, it is challenging and necessary to design an energy-efficient mechanism with the consideration of the characteristics of WBSNs. Motivated by the existing work, in this chapter, we firstly propose an energy-efficient leader election (EELE) mechanism for WBSNs.

Moreover, the reliability is a stringent requirement on medical applications closely related to human's health. Due to the high path loss on human body, it has been justified that directed communication with the sink is inefficient and unreliable for far nodes [3]. Besides, the packet error rate probability and the related outage probability of each on-body link are related with the body movement and posture. It is observed that cooperative transmission scheme achieves a performance enhancement in terms of packet error rate versus transmitted power [4]. Furthermore, two-hop cooperative communication was adopted in IEEE 802.15.6 standard [5] as an option to overcome significantly the path loss in WBSNs. Inspired by the aforementioned existing analysis, we then come up with a reliable and energy-efficient leader election (REELE) algorithm for WBSNs, subsequently.

## 2.1.2   Summary of Contributions

In this chapter, we investigate the reliable and energy-efficient leader election algorithms for WBSNs. The main contributions of this chapter are articulated as follows:

- Firstly, we partition a WBSN into regions as the same definition as the cluster to manage sensors efficiently and introduce the network model.
- Secondly, a distance-aware hybrid communication approach is introduced which benefits to relieve the burden of the far nodes and the leader. And we develop a distributed leader election algorithm where the utility function considers the influence of the location and the residual energy of the nodes.

- Then, we model the reliability as the probability of successful communication and formulate the total energy consumption model. A reliable and energy-efficient communication strategy is proposed. Correspondingly, we propose a distributed algorithm by jointly considering reliability, residual energy, and total energy consumption to select the optimal leader in each region and analyze its complexity.
- Finally, we comprehensively evaluate the performance of EELE and REELE by extensive simulation. And the simulation results demonstrate the effectiveness and efficiency of EELE and REELE in terms of network lifetime, energy conservation, throughput as well as the reliability compared with existing solutions.

## 2.2  Related Work

In recent years, for the primary importance of energy conservation on network longevity, considerable researchers have proved that cluster-based is an efficient scheme in increasing network lifetime and scalability of WSNs [6, 7]. In cluster-based schemes, there are two types of nodes in one cluster, one cluster head or cluster leader and several cluster members. Cluster members monitor data periodically and send it to the cluster head. Cluster head aggregates data from all its members, compresses the data to eliminate redundancy, and transmits the compressed data to base station. Thus, in cluster-based protocol, the energy consumption can be reduced by stipulating that only a small fraction of the nodes are allowed to communicate with the base station.

Cluster head selection has very significant impact on the energy efficiency of the clustering protocol given the load concentration at those nodes. To effectively elect the leader for each cluster, Heinzelamn et al. study a low energy adaptive cluster hierarchy (LEACH) protocol for wireless microsensor networks in [1]. In LEACH, each node have the same probability to be cluster head. Once the nodes have elected themselves to be cluster heads, they must broadcast an advertisement message to let all the other nodes in the network know that they have chosen this role for the current round. Each non-cluster head node determines its cluster by choosing the cluster head that requires the minimum communication energy for this round. After each node has decided to which cluster it belongs, it must inform the cluster head that it will be a member of the cluster. So that, LEACH provides a balance of energy consumption through a random rotation of cluster heads among all nodes in the networks. However, a cluster head expends much more energy to transmit the data to the base station. The nodes with low energy will die more rapidly than that with high energy. Consider the impact of cluster head position on variance of overall energy consumption, the authors [8] have proposed an enhancement of low energy adaptive clustering hierarchy (e-health) which ensures a node with higher mean value of remain energy and low variance can be elected as a cluster head. The basic idea is to minimize the variance of remaining energy of the nodes so as to maximize the lifetime of the network. Therefore, the nodes with the highest remaining energy and the lowest energy variance consumption become the cluster heads with high probability. The additional variance parameter takes into account energy consumption dispersion if the considered node is elected as a cluster head. The dispersion highly depends on the relative positioning of the node to the base station.

Besides, a hybrid energy-efficient distributed cluster (HEED) approach is proposed for ad hoc sensor networks in [2] where the cluster heads are chosen based on two important parameters: residual energy and intra-cluster communication cost. Initially, each node probabilistically becomes a tentative cluster head depending on its remaining energy. The final cluster heads are selected according to the intra-cluster communication cost which reflects the node degree or node's proximity to the neighbor. For the non-cluster head nodes, they should go through several iterations until they find the cluster head that they can transmit to with the least transmission power. Therefore, HEED provides a uniform cluster head distribution across the network and better load balancing by considering a hybrid of energy and communication cost. However, several iterations involved in cluster formation and knowledge of the entire network can lead to large overhead cost. Thus, the nodes which are near the base station may die earlier.

In [9], the authors have proposed and evaluated two novel clustering-based protocols for heterogeneous WSNs, which are called single-hop energy-efficient clustering protocol (S-EECP) and multi-hop energy-efficient clustering protocol (M-EECP). In S-EECP the cluster heads are elected by a weighted probability based on the ratio between residual energy of each node and average energy of the network. The nodes with high initial energy and residual energy will have more chance to be elected as cluster heads than those with low energy. Whereas in M-EECP, after the election of cluster heads, member nodes communicate with their respective cluster head by using single-hop communication. The cluster heads collect the data from their member nodes and transfer them to the base station via multi-hop communication approach. Therefore, S-EECP and M-EECP protocols can extend network lifetime and consume less energy to balance energy consumption among cluster heads.

However, due to the typical features of WBSNs, such as the limited energy resources and special communication medium, the existing protocols for the large-scale WSNs are not exactly applicable to the WBSNs. Therefore, it is challenging and necessary to design an energy-efficient mechanism with the consideration of the characteristics of WBSNs.

On the other hand, due to the unique properties of WBSNs with distinct channel characteristics and very small scale, the reliable communication is necessary to guarantee, especially for the medical surgery monitoring applications closely related to human's health. To the best of our knowledge, there is only limited work on the network reliability for WBSNs. Due to the high path loss [3] on human body, the authors have investigated an energy-efficient cooperative relay selection scheme in [10]. With a realistic nonlinear energy consumption model, they have proposed that direct communication is preferable for conserving energy when the transmitter and receiver are located on the same side of the human body without significant

**Table 2.1**  Comparison of the clustering protocols

| Protocols | CH selection | Energy balanced | Energy efficiency | Reliability |
|-----------|--------------|-----------------|-------------------|-------------|
| LEACH     | Random       | No              | Low               | No          |
| e-LEACH   | Random       | Good            | Low               | No          |
| HEED      | Probability  | Good            | High              | No          |
| S/M-EECP  | Probability  | Good            | Low               | No          |
| EELE      | Probability  | Very good       | Very high         | No          |
| REELE     | Probability  | Very good       | Very high         | Yes         |

path loss. However, at a suitable relay location and with large transmission distance, the cooperative communication can achieve a significant improvement on energy efficiency when the transmitter and receiver are located on the different sides of the human body. In [11], the authors have analyzed the outage probability performance in three transmission schemes, i.e., direct transmission, single-relay cooperative, and multi-relay cooperative. In order to minimize the energy consumption, the optimal power allocation problem with the constraint of targeted outage probability is proposed, where the impact of posture and movement of human body on the wireless channel is considered. And the cooperative communication has been demonstrated that it can help to reduce the outage probability and to improve the energy efficiency for most of the typical channel quality due to the fixed transceiver locations on human body. Moreover, the packet error rate probability and the related outage probability of each on-body link were investigated in [4]. It is observed that cooperative transmission scheme achieves a performance enhancement in terms of packet error rate versus transmitted power. Furthermore, two-hop cooperative communication is adopted in IEEE 802.15.6 standard [5] as an option to overcome significantly the path loss in WBSNs.

Motivated by the aforementioned existing analysis, we argue that a novel study based on cluster topology and cooperative communication is called for in order to improve the network reliability and prolong the network lifetime for WBSNs. Therefore, we will firstly propose an energy-efficient leader election mechanism where a WBSN is partitioned into several regions and a distance-aware hybrid communication approach and distributed leader election algorithm are introduced. Then, we extend it to a reliable and energy-efficient leader election algorithm, where the reliability is modeled as the probability of successful communication and the optimal leader is elected by jointly considering reliability, residual energy, and total energy consumption in each region. For clearness, Table 2.1 shows the comparison between the existing clustering protocols and our proposed protocols.

## 2.3  Network Model

Cluster head selection has very significant impact on the energy efficiency of the clustering protocols. However, due to the unique properties of WBSNs with distinct channel characteristics and very small scale, the existing energy-efficient cluster head election mechanisms for large-scale WSNs are inadequate if they are applied to WBSNs directly. Therefore, we propose a set of energy-efficient leader election mechanisms for WBSNs in this chapter.

Inspired by the cluster-based topology and the native symmetry of the human body, we partition a WBSN network into $M$ logical regions as the same definition as the clusters to achieve high energy efficiency and enhance the network scalability. In each region, there are $I$ energy limited sensor nodes which can be classified into $K$ types based on their individual application functions. For convenient distinction, each sensor node is assigned a region identification number (*RID*), a type identification number (*TID*), and a node identification number (*NID*), respectively. Definitely, the region set in a WBSN is $R = \{r_1, \ldots, r_m, \ldots, r_M\}$, where $|R| = M$ and $r_m$ represents the $m$-th region. Correspondingly, the type set is $T = \{t_1, \ldots, t_k, \ldots, t_K\}$, where $|T| = K$ and $t_k$ is indicated the $k$-th type node. Also, the node set is $N = \{n_1, \ldots, n_i, \ldots, n_I\}$, where $|N| = I$ and the $i$-th sensor is described as $n_i$. Consequently, we can use the triple $\langle r_m, t_k, n_i \rangle$ to uniquely indicate the $i$-th sensor of the $k$-th type in the $m$-th region. Note that we use the terms of "node" and "sensor node" interchangeably to refer to the same WBSN entity.

Besides, we make the following reasonable assumptions about the nodes and the network model for analytical tractability:

- All nodes are stationary after the deployment. And they also know the relevant information about themselves, such as the location and the real-time residual energy.
- All nodes are of the same sensing and computation capability. And they always have packets to send during their active periods.
- One and only one leader is elected like the cluster head in each region to manage and schedule other nodes, correspondingly the other nodes are the normal members.
- The leader must directly communicate with the sink which is located in the center of the body, while the normal nodes can transmit directly with enough power to reach the sink if needed.
- During the active periods, the leader firstly aggregates packets from normal members into one packet of fixed size and transforms it to the sink. Note that the leader is the relay in cooperative communication to help others to transfer their packets to the sink.

In WBSNs, most of the devices are attached on human body, so the communications between nodes and the sink occur along the surface of the human body which contributes attenuation to radio signal. As we are just interested in the energy consumption of the communication, which is much larger than the energy used for sensing, we ignore the latter in this dissertation. According to the radio hardware energy dissipation model shown in [12], the energy consumption model for transmitting and receiving $l$-bits data over distance $d$ is

$$\begin{cases} E_{Tx}(l, d, n) & = l E_{Txelec} + l \epsilon_{amp}(n) d^n, \\ E_{Rx}(l) & = l E_{Rxelec}, \end{cases} \tag{2.1}$$

where $E_{Txelec}$ and $E_{Rxelec}$ are the energy dissipated by the radio to run the circuitry for the transmitter and the receiver, respectively, and $\epsilon_{amp}$ is the energy for the transmission amplifier. $d$ is the distance between the transmitter and the receiver, whereas $n$ represents the path loss coefficient ($n = 3.11$ for the LOS (line-of-signal) channel and $n = 5.9$ for the NLOS (non-line-of-signal) channel). Particularly, if one node is elected as the final leader, it will aggregate the original packets from the normal nodes into one single length-fixed packet and then send it to the sink, so the leader will consume extra $E_{DA}$ energy for the data aggregation.

## 2.4  Proposed Energy-Efficient Leader Election Mechanism

In this section, we develop an energy-efficient leader election mechanism, called EELE. Firstly, the hybrid communication mode is introduced with the consideration of distance. We then propose a distributed leader election algorithm based on utility function and present the complexity analysis of this algorithm. Subsequently, we evaluate the performance of the proposed EELE mechanism and compare it with two other schemes derived from LEACH [1] and HEED [2] which are the most classical energy-efficient mechanisms: LEACH-Analogous (LEACH-A) and HEED-Analogous (HEED-A).

### 2.4.1  Energy Consumption-Based Hybrid Communication Strategy

In wireless communications, nodes can adopt direct communication or cooperative communication. Under the direct communication, each node can send its data directly to the sink in WBSNs. But if the node is far away from the sink, the direct communication will require a large amount of transmission power as shown in Eq. (2.1), which will quickly drain the battery of the far node and shorten the network lifetime. Therefore, the cooperative communication is exploited, in which the packets from the far nodes can be relayed to the sink by an intermediate node, so that the energy dissipation of the far node will be reduced. However, the cooperative communication is not suitable for the nodes close to the sink. If a closer node also employs cooperative communication, it will not only consume its own energy, but also consume the energy of the intermediate node.

Motivated by the aforementioned analysis, we can draw a conclusion that the direct communication is more energy-efficient for the closer node, while the cooperative communication is more energy-efficient for the farther node. Therefore, a hybrid communication mode which is more suitable for WBSNs is developed as follows. In each region, there is only one intermediate node which is in the term of "leader" afterwards. Correspondingly, the other nodes will be in the term of "normal node." The leader will aggregate the packets from the normal nodes and transfer it to the sink in direct communication. For a normal node, it can choose the communication mode according to the distance ($D_1$) between it and the sink and the distance ($D_2$) between the leader and the sink. If $D_1 > D_2$, it will choose cooperative communication mode. Otherwise, the direct communication mode will be selected.

Consequently, when direct communication mode is used the leader is relieved of its relaying burden for nodes closer to the sink. Similarly, when cooperative communication mode is used the nodes far from the sink are relieved of their burden of long range transmissions to the sink. Thus by adaptively adjusting communication mode it is probable to conserve energy consumption and obtain a uniform load distribution.

### 2.4.2  Leader Election Algorithm

Considering the WBSNs characteristics, one tentative leader is randomly chosen from each type. Let $g_k$ define the number of the nodes falling into the $k$-th type, satisfying $\sum_{k=1}^{K} g_k = I$. If node $n_i$ is affiliated with the $k$-th type, it will compete to be a tentative leader with the probability $P_i(t)$ at time $t$,

$$P_i(t) = 1/g_k. \tag{2.2}$$

So the expected number of the tentative leader per round is $K$. Then the optimal one among them is elected to be the final leader according to the utility function. In order to balance the task of becoming as the leader, the utility function is related with the residual energy and the distance between the node and the sink. For node $n_i$ the utility function at time $t$ is

$$UF(i, t) = \left( \frac{R_0}{d(i, sink)} \right)^{\alpha} \cdot \left( \frac{RE(i, t)}{E_0} \right)^{1-\alpha}, \tag{2.3}$$

where $R_0$ is the region communication radius, and $d(i, sink)$ denotes the distance between node $n_i$ and the sink. $E_0$ and $RE(i, t)$ are the initial energy and the residual energy of node $n_i$ at time $t$, respectively. $\alpha \in [0, 1]$ is the weight that indicates the preference for the distance or the residual energy. Particularly, when $\alpha = 0$, it implies the residual energy is the only criterion to be the final leader. And when $\alpha = 1$, it means that the node closest to the sink will be the final leader.

In the proposed algorithm, an arbitrary tentative leader $n_i$ maintains a set $C_{ni}$ of its competitors. A competitor $n_j$ is also a tentative leader with the same $RID$

as $n_i$ but different *TID* from $n_i$. Whether a tentative leader becomes as the final leader successfully depends on its utility function. If one node wins as the leader, the other normal nodes will act as its members. A formal description of the disposed algorithm is shown in Algorithm 1.

---

**Algorithm 1** Leader election algorithm

1: $\mu \leftarrow RAND(0, 1)$;
2: **if** $\mu < P_i(t)$ and $RE(i, t) > 0$ **then**
3:     $TentativeLeader \leftarrow TRUE$;
4: **end if**
5: **if** $TentativeLeader = TRUE$ **then**
6:     $CompeteMsg(RID, TID, NID, d(i, sink), RE)$;
7: **end if**
8: On receiving a COMPETE_MSG from node $n_j$;
9: **if** $RID_i = RID_j$ and $TID_i \neq TID_j$ **then**
10:     add $n_j$ to $C_{ni}$;
11: **end if**
12: **if** $C_{ni} \neq \varnothing$ **then**
13:     **if** $UF(n_i) > UF(n_j), \forall n_j \in C_{ni}$ **then**
14:         $LeaderMsg(NID, d(i, sink), RE)$;
15:     **else if** $UF(n_i) = UF(n_j)$ **then**
16:         **if** $RE(i, t) \geq RE(j, t)$ **then**
17:             $LeaderMsg(NID, d(i, sink), RE)$;
18:         **else**
19:             $QuitMsg(TID, NID)$;
20:         **end if**
21:     **end if**
22:     On receiving a LEADER_MSG from node $n_j$ ;
23:     **if** $\forall n_j \in C_{ni}$ **then**
24:         $QuitMsg(TID, NID)$;
25:     **end if**
26:     On receiving a QUIT_MSG from node $n_j$;
27:     **if** $\forall n_j \in C_{ni}$ **then**
28:         remove $n_j$ from $C_{ni}$;
29:     **end if**
30: **end if**

---

In the leader election algorithm, the broadcast radius of every control message is $R_0$, thus $n_i$ can receive all message from the nodes in its $C_{ni}$. Initially, several nodes are elected to be tentative leaders with the probability $P_i(t)$. And the other nodes keep sleeping until the final leader is selected. If one node becomes the tentative node successfully, it will broadcast a COMPETE_MSG message which contains its *RID*, *TID*, *NID*, and *RE* as lines 5–7 in Algorithm 1. Then, if node $n_i$ receives a COMPETE_MSG from node $n_j$ with the same region number, it will add $n_j$ to its competitor set $C_{ni}$. After the competitor set has been formed in lines 8–11, each tentative leader checks its utility function and makes a decision whether it can act as the final leader as in lines 12–21. Once $n_i$ finds its utility function more than that of the other nodes in $C_{ni}$, it will win as the leader successfully and will broadcast

a LEADER_MSG. In case of the same utility value, we choose the node with more
$RE$. Otherwise, if node $n_i$ receives a LEADER_MSG from $n_j$ in lines 22–25, it will
give up the competition immediately, and inform other nodes by a QUIT_MSG. Or
else, it will remove $n_j$ from its $C_{ni}$ once receiving a QUIT_MSG from $n_j$.

According to Algorithm 1, the leader election process is message driven, thus we
discuss its complexity below.

**Lemma 2.1** *The control overhead complexity of the leader election algorithm is*
$O(I)$, *where $I$ is the number of nodes.*

*Proof* Observing EELE, every node sends out a few quite short control messages each round without iteration. At the start of the leader election phase,
$\sum_{k=1}^{K} g_k P_i(t){=}K$ tentative leaders are produced and each of them broadcasts a
COMPETE_MSG. As described aforementioned, $P_i(t)$ determines the number of
tentative leaders. Then, each of them either broadcasts a LEADER_MSG to act as a
final leader or broadcasts a QUIT_MSG to be a normal node. For only one leader is
elected in one region, they send out one LEADER_MSG and $(K - 1)$ QUIT_MSGs.
Once the leader has been elected, the normal nodes will decide their communication
mode and inform the leader by a short control message. Thus, the messages add up
to $2K + 2(I - 1)$ per round. Since $K < I$, the total asymptotic order of the control
overhead is $O(I)$.                                                              □

*Remark* The number of nodes in a WBSN is extremely limited by nature of the
network. Consequently, Lemma 2.1 verifies the message overhead of Algorithm 1
is very small.

### 2.4.3  Energy-Efficient Leader Election Mechanism

A fundamental problem in WBSNs is to maximize the network lifetime under given
energy constraints. In order to conserve the energy and ensure that all nodes die
approximately at the same time, the operation of EELE is divided into *rounds* to
make the nodes in different regions wake up alternately as shown in Fig. 2.1. After
the initial phase, each round begins with the set-up phase when the leader is elected,

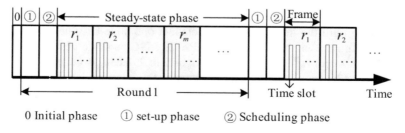

**Fig. 2.1** The time line of EELE operation

followed by the scheduling phase. At last, the network accesses into the steady-state phase when the nodes transmit packets to the sink once a communication mode is chosen. The time line is shown in Fig. 2.1. The following subsections describe the operation procedure of EELE in details.

**Initial Phase** Initially, the deployment is established using recommendation of medical institutes and some optimal deployment methods [12]. Then, the sink broadcasts a "hello" message including its location to all nodes. After receiving the message, each node can compute and store the approximate distance to the sink based on the received signal. Subsequently, each node establishes an information table which consists of its *RID*, *TID*, *NID*, *RE* and its distance to the sink. At the end of each round, the nodes update their residual energy immediately.

**Set-Up Phase** In this phase, the main task is to elect the leader in each region. All nodes are initialized with an equal amount of energy, and they always send the data about the physiological parameters during the active period. According to the Algorithm 1, the tentative leaders will compete for the final leader. Simultaneously, the other nodes turn into sleep state. Once the leaders have been eventually settled, they must inform the sink and all the normal nodes of their roles as the leaders for the current round. Meanwhile, the sleeping nodes must wake up and receive the final message LEADER_MSG. Each normal node determines its communication mode in this round and informs the leader by sending a short message. Then the leader aggregates the messages from all normal nodes into one single packet, and transfers it to the sink.

**Scheduling Phase** After receiving the aggregative messages from the $M$ leaders, the sink sets up a TDMA schedule and transmits it to each leader. On receiving the TDMA schedule, each leader sets up a sub-TDMA schedule and informs its members. Through the sub-TDMA schedule, the leader manages only one node for each type to work while the others to get into sleep status and ensure that every active normal node just transmits once per round. Subsequently, the steady-state operation can begin.

**Steady-State Phase** The steady-state phase is divided into frames which are assigned to the different regions based on the TDMA schedule. And each frame is further partitioned into time slots which are assigned to nodes based on the sub-TDMA schedule. Finally, each node sends its data to the sink or the leader during its assigned time slot, respectively.

The operation flowchart of the aforementioned EELE mechanism on a node is shown in Fig. 2.2.

### 2.4.4  Performance Evaluation

In the simulation, we assess the performance of EELE in terms of:

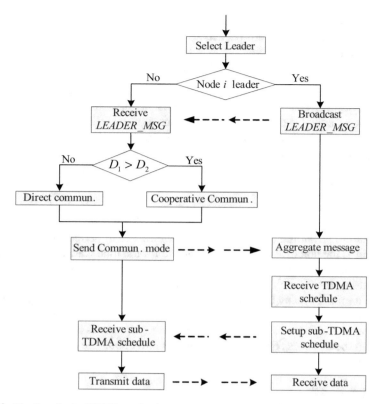

**Fig. 2.2** The flowchart of EELE mechanism

- *Network lifetime*: Lifetime is the vital criterion for evaluating the performance of WBSNs, which is defined as the time until the first node or the last node dies.
- *Energy characteristics*: To verify the effectiveness and efficiency of EELE on the energy conservation, the average residual energy and the energy efficiency will be evaluated. The definition of the later is the ratio of the total received data to the total energy consumption.
- *Throughput*: Throughput is defined as the average receiving data successfully per round.

According to the symmetry of human body and the location of the sink node, a WBSN is partitioned into four equal regions as shown in Fig. 2.3. Due to the nature of the network, the number of nodes in a WBSN is limited in the range of 20–50. Consequently, 10 sensor nodes are deployed in each region and categorized into five types based on their monitoring function, separately. And the detailed simulation parameters are given in Table 2.2, where the radio parameters of the Nordic nRF2401 transceiver [12] are employed. Moreover, every simulation results are the average of 100 independent experiments.

**Fig. 2.3** Sensor location

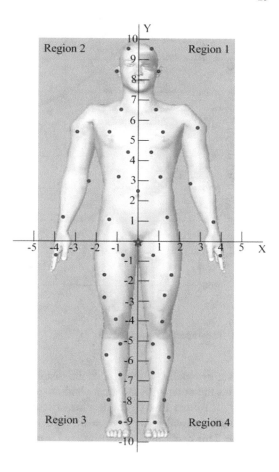

**Table 2.2** Simulation settings

| Parameter | Setting | Parameter | Setting |
|-----------|---------|-----------|---------|
| One region coverage | (0, 0) (50, 100) | $E_{Txelec}$ | 16.7 nJ/bit |
| Packet size | 4000 bits | $E_{Rxelec}$ | 36.1 nJ/bit |
| Initial energy | 0.1 J | $E_{DA}$ | 5 nJ/bit/signal |
| Shadowing Std | $\sigma = 6.2$ | $\epsilon_{amp}(n)$ | 1.97 nJ/(bit m$^n$), ($n = 3.11$) |

In EELE mechanism, we choose the leaders through the maximum utility function with the residual energy and the location of the node taken into consideration. As described in Sect. 2.4.2, $\alpha$ determines the proportional factor of the residual energy and the distance, which means the preference for the distance or the residual energy when electing the leader. Thus we need adopt an optimal value to prolong the network lifetime.

The relation between $\alpha$ and the network lifetime is shown in Fig. 2.4. When $\alpha$ varies from 0 to 1, the influence of the residual energy on the utility function

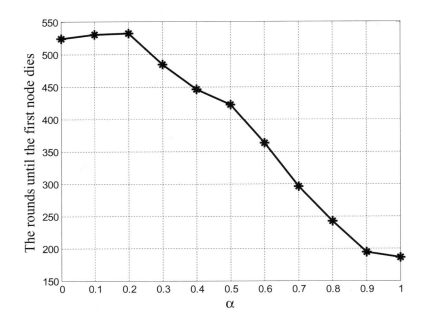

**Fig. 2.4** The impact of $\alpha$ on lifetime

decreases gradually, while that of the distance increases. Particularly, when $\alpha = 0$, it implies the node with the most residual energy is elected as the leader. And when $\alpha = 1$, it means that the node closest to the sink will be the leader. Obviously, there is an optimal value of $\alpha = 0.2$ when the network can achieve the maximum lifetime. This result indicates the energy is more prioritized when electing the leader. Therefore, we use $\alpha = 0.2$ in the following simulations.

In Figs. 2.5 and 2.6, we assess the network lifetime in terms of the dead nodes and the percentage of remaining alive nodes. As shown in Fig. 2.5, EELE mechanism clearly improves network lifetime over LEACH-A and HEED-A. Furthermore, Fig. 2.6 shows the total number of nodes that remain alive over the simulation time. In EELE there are quite more alive nodes than those in others at the same time. Specifically, the first node died at the 529th round in EELE which are 34 and 92 rounds later than that in HEED-A and that in LEACH-A, respectively. Moreover, there are still 90% nodes alive in EELE when all nodes are dead in both HEED-A and LEACH-A.

The reason is that every node has the equal probability to become the leader in LEACH-A. Once the node with rather less residual energy is elected as the leader, it will be dead easily and fast. While in HEED-A the far nodes have a bigger probability to become leaders, resulting in the more energy dissipated. But this is avoided in EELE since the far node will be a leader if and only if its residual energy is considerably larger than that of the near one, and this obviously reduces the probability of the far node to become the leader. Even if the far node competes

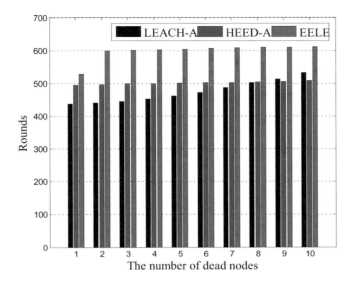

**Fig. 2.5**  The time until a given number of nodes die

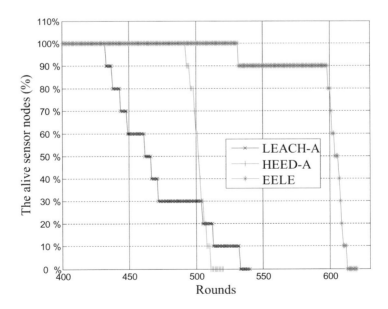

**Fig. 2.6**  The percent of the alive nodes over time

as the leader, the closer node can communicate directly with the sink in EELE, which alleviates the burden of the leader. The above results shows EELE can indeed efficiently prolong the network lifetime.

In this part, we investigate the average residual energy per node and the energy efficiency. Fifty rounds of simulations are sampled and the results are shown in Figs. 2.7 and 2.8. EELE achieves more residual energy and higher energy efficiency than the others.

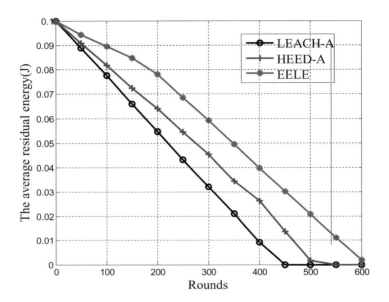

**Fig. 2.7** The average residual energy over time

**Fig. 2.8** The network energy efficiency over time

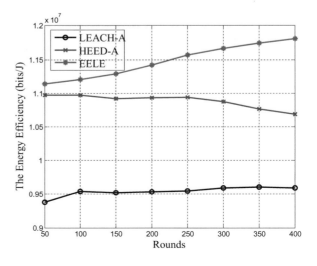

In LEACH-A and HEED-A, all the packets of normal nodes must be sent to the
leader and then the leader transfers them to the sink. But a far node can compete as
the leader with the same probability as a closer node in LEACH-A. As also, a far
one competes as the leader with an increasing probability as the simulation runs in
HEED-A. Once the far one wins as the leader, the closer ones must transmit their
packets to it. As a result, the leader has to consume more energy to transfer the same
data over a longer distance.

Differently, EELE scheme lowers the probability of a far node to be the leader
unless it has obviously much more residual energy. Moreover, the adopted hybrid
communication mode benefits to relieve the burden of the far nodes and the leaders.
Accordingly, the energy efficiency of EELE increases slightly as the operation of
the WBSN. Therefore, the energy efficiency of EELE is much better than that of
LEACH-A and HEED-A.

As shown in Fig. 2.9, with the value of the initial enery varied, the EELE achieves
the highest throughput. Accurately, EELE outperforms LEACH-A and HEED-A
over up to 51.7% and 33.7%, respectively. It is the superiority of EELE mechanism
in the effectiveness and energy efficiency on energy conservation that contributes to
more delivered packets.

According to the above analysis, we can draw a conclusion that EELE is more
suitable for the energy constraint and small-scale network such as WBSNs.

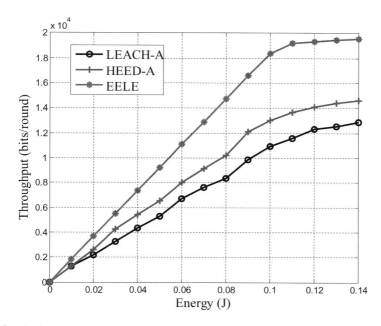

**Fig. 2.9**  The throughput over different initial energy

## 2.5   Proposed Reliable and Energy-Efficient Leader Election Mechanism

In this section, we present a reliable and energy-efficient leader election mechanism, called REELE, for WBSNs to elect the region leader based on the reliability and energy consumption analysis and further analyze its complexity and the performance in terms of network lifetime, energy characteristics, and reliability.

### 2.5.1   Reliability Model

Due to high pass loss around the human body, it has been justified that nodes in the same side of the body can communicate more reliably with each other than with nodes in the other side [10]. This observation prompts us that communication should happen between the nodes in the same side of the body, which also verifies the feasibility of the proposed partitioning idea. Therefore, we propose a reliable and energy-efficient leader election algorithm for WBSNs based on the same network model as described in Sect. 2.4 and the same sensors deployment as shown in Fig. 2.3.

In order to develop the reliability in WBSNs, we firstly need to model the path loss between the transmitting and receiving antennas as a function of the distance $d$. In our analysis, we use the following semi-empirical formula which is expressed in decibel and based on the Friis formula [3]

$$PL_{\mathrm{dB}}(d) = PL_{0,\mathrm{dB}} + 10 \cdot n \cdot \log(d/d_0), \tag{2.4}$$

where $P_{0,\mathrm{dB}}$ is the path loss in dB at a reference distance $d_0$ (10 cm in this chapter) and $n$ is the path loss exponent which equals 2 in free space.

In practice, there exists shadow fading defined as the variation of the local mean around the path loss. To guarantee the reliable communication, it is essential to account for this factor. Thereby, the total path loss becomes a random variable defined as

$$PL = PL_{\mathrm{dB}} + PL_s, \tag{2.5}$$

where $PL_{\mathrm{dB}}$ is the value predicted by the path loss model as Eq. (2.4), and the shadowing component $PL_s$ is represented by a zero-mean Gaussian random variable $X_{\sigma,\mathrm{dB}}$ with standard deviation $\sigma$ in dB.

Thus the signal strength $P_{r,\mathrm{dB}}^{j}$ at a receiver $n_j$ from a transmitter $n_i$ with transmitting power $P_{s,\mathrm{dB}}^{i}$ over a distance $d_{ij}$ can be computed as

$$P_{r,\mathrm{dB}}^{j}(d_{ij}) = P_{s,\mathrm{dB}}^{i} - PL_{\mathrm{dB}}(d_{ij}) - X_{\sigma,\mathrm{dB}}. \tag{2.6}$$

In this dissertation, we evaluate the reliability from the perspective of the received signal strength at the receiver as done in wireless communication. If the signal strength $P_{r,\text{dB}}^{j}$ is higher than a certain threshold $P_{th}$, the received packet can be acknowledged. Conversely, the link is interrupted and the unreliable communication will happen. As a result, the reliability can be modeled as the probability $p(d_{ij})$ of successful communication between two nodes $n_i$ and $n_j$, which is formulated as follows:

$$p(d_{ij}) = \Pr[P_{r,\text{dB}}^{j}(d_{ij}) > P_{th}] = \Pr[X_{\sigma,\text{dB}} + \mu(d_{ij}) < 0], \qquad (2.7)$$

where the left part of the second inequality can be seen as a normal distribution with the standard deviation $\sigma$ and the mean $\mu(d_{ij})$ shown as follows:

$$\mu(d_{ij}) = -P_{s,\text{dB}}^{i} + PL_{0,\text{dB}} + 10n\log_{10}(d_{ij}/d_0) + P_{th}. \qquad (2.8)$$

Consequently, the probability in Eq. (2.7) can be rewritten as:

$$p(d_{ij}) = \frac{1}{\sqrt{2\pi}\sigma} \int_{-\infty}^{0} \exp\left[-\frac{(t-\mu(d_{ij}))^2}{2\sigma^2}\right] dt = \frac{1}{2} - \frac{1}{2}\text{erf}\left(\frac{\mu(d_{ij})}{\sqrt{2\pi}\sigma}\right), \qquad (2.9)$$

where erf() is the standard cumulative error function. It is clear that the reliable communication probability also depends on transmitting power $P_{s,\text{dB}}^{i}$ and receiving threshold $P_{th}$. In IEEE 802.15.6 WBSNs standard [5], the former can be set from $-25$ to $0\,\text{dBm}$. And the latter is defined by the parameters of the receiver. For instance, if the noise floor is $-90\,\text{dBm}$ and the required signal-to-noise ratio is at least $20\,\text{dB}$, $P_{th}$ can be set as $-70\,\text{dBm}$.

Accordingly, based on the region topology and cooperative communication, we develop a reliable and energy-efficient communication strategy suitable for WBSNs in the following subsection.

## 2.5.2 Reliable and Energy-Efficient Communication Strategy

Although cooperative communication scheme has been proved more energy effi-cient in many cases, it is not applicable to all nodes specially for the small scale WBSNs. Moreover, the network reliability is overlooked in many studies. Therefore, by considering energy efficiency and network reliability jointly we propose a novel communication strategy which is applicable to WBSNs.

Here, we detail the novel communication strategy. Once the only one leader is elected, correspondingly the other nodes are the normal members in each region. As an assumption, the leader must adopt direct communication with the sink. If a node $n_k$ is elected as the leader, a normal node $n_i$ will determine whether or not to implement cooperative communication by the following rules: (1) It firstly judges whether its distance to the sink $d_{i,s}$ is larger than that between the leader and the sink $d_{k,s}$; and (2) it compares the reliability probability $p(d_{i,k}) \cdot p(d_{k,s})$ of the cooperative communication with that $p(d_{i,s})$ of the direct communication. If the inequalities $d_{i,s} > d_{k,s}$ and $p(d_{i,k}) \cdot p(d_{k,s}) > p(d_{i,s})$ hold, the node will choose cooperative communication. Otherwise, the direct communication is adopted.

The reason for the design is twofold. For the far nodes, the direct communication with the sink requires a large transmission energy, which quickly drains the battery and shorten the network lifetime. Moreover, the large distance also results in the increase of outage probability. Therefore, cooperative communication is necessary to reduce the energy dissipation and to enhance the reliability of the far nodes. However, for the nodes close to the sink, it is obvious that more energy of both nodes and the leader will be consumed if the leader is farther from the sink. In other words, cooperative communication is not beneficial for the short distance communication. Besides, the reliability of the source–leader–sink link will be deteriorated instead of improvement in this case. Thus, the direct communication is preferable conversely.

Consequently, when direct communication is preferred by the close nodes, the leader is relieved of its relaying burden. While cooperative communication can offer more advantage in alleviating the long distance transmissions and improving the reliability for the far nodes. Thus adaptively adjusting communication mode can significantly boost network performance.

### 2.5.3  Total Energy Consumption Model

In order to analyze the energy consumption, we use the same energy model as shown in Eq. (2.1). The leader aggregates the packets original from the normal nodes into one single length-fixed packet and will transform it to the sink, so the leader will consume extra $E_{DA}$ energy for the data aggregation.

Before calculating the total energy consumption, we first introduce the following notations. Let node $n_k$ be the leader in the $m$-th region. Define an indication variable as follows:

$$R_{k,m} = \begin{cases} 1 & \text{if } n_k \text{ is the leader in region } r_m, \\ 0 & \text{otherwise,} \end{cases} \qquad (2.10)$$

which is subjected to $\sum_{m=1}^{M} \sum_{k=1}^{N} R_{k,m} = M$.

As for normal nodes, they employ the proposed reliable and energy-efficient communication strategy. Let $D_{i,m}$ indicate whether node $n_i$ chooses the direct communication

$$D_{i,m} = \begin{cases} 1 & \text{if } n_i \text{ selects direct commun. and } n_i \text{ is in the } m\text{-th region, } i \in N, i \neq k, \\ 0 & \text{otherwise.} \end{cases}$$

$$(2.11)$$

Correspondingly, a variable indicating whether node $n_i$ chooses the cooperative communication can be described as

$$C_{i,m} = \begin{cases} 1 & \text{if } n_i \text{ selects cooperative commun. and } n_i \\ & \text{is in the } m\text{-th region, } i \in N, i \neq k, \\ 0 & \text{otherwise.} \end{cases} \qquad (2.12)$$

Thus, the sum of nodes choosing the cooperative communication in the $m$-th region can be expressed as $B_m = \sum_{i=1}^{N} C_{i,m}$.

Given the above notations and energy consumption model, the total energy consumption of region $r_m$ can be separated into four parts: (1) energy consumption of direct transmission from the normal nodes to the sink, $\sum_{i\in N, i\neq k} D_{i,m} \cdot E_{Tx}$; (2) energy consumption of cooperative transmission from the normal nodes to the leader, $\sum_{i\in N, i\neq k} C_{i,m} \cdot E_{Tx}$; (3) energy consumption of the leader used to receive and aggregate the packets from other nodes, $\sum_{k\in N} R_{k,m}(E_{Rx} \cdot B_m + E_{DA})$; (4) energy consumption of transmission from the leader to the sink, $\sum_{k\in N} R_{k,m} \cdot E_{Tx}$. As a result, the total energy consumption can be derived as follows:

$$\begin{aligned} E_{total} = & \sum_{i\in N, i\neq k} D_{i,m} \left( l \cdot E_{Txelec} + l \cdot \varepsilon_{amp} d_{i,s}^n \right) \\ & + \sum_{i\in N, i\neq k} C_{i,m} \left( l \cdot E_{Txelec} + l \cdot \varepsilon_{amp} d_{i,k}^n \right) \\ & + \sum_{k\in N} R_{k,m} \left( l \cdot E_{Rxelec} \cdot B_m + E_{DA} \right) \\ & + \sum_{k\in N} R_{k,m} \left( l \cdot E_{Txelec} + l \cdot \varepsilon_{amp} d_{k,s}^n \right). \end{aligned} \qquad (2.13)$$

### 2.5.4  Reliable Leader Election Algorithm

The goal of REELE algorithm is to select a best leader in one region to reduce the energy consumption and improve the reliability. On account of the scarce battery capacity and the importance of reliability, REELE primarily screens nodes based on the residual energy and reliability. Then the total energy consumption as the third condition is considered to prolong network lifetime. A formal description is shown in Algorithm 2 for an arbitrary node $n_i$.

In REELE algorithm, we assume that nodes in the same region can receive all control messages from other nodes and know their locations by an ideal neighbor discovery process which is not our focus. Before executing the algorithm, each node initially establishes and updates an information table consisting of its *RID*, *NID*,

---

**Algorithm 2** Leader election algorithm

---

**I. Initialize**

  1: Infor.Table $\leftarrow$ ($RID$, $NID$, $Location$, $E_0$, $E_i(t)$)
  2: $p_i(t) \leftarrow$ max($E_i(t)/E_0$, $p_{min}$)
  3: $p(d_{i,s}) \leftarrow$ equation (2.9)
  4: be_Tentative_Leader $\leftarrow$ FALSE
  5: be_Final_Leader $\leftarrow$ FALSE

**II. Main Processing**

  1: **if** Random (0,1) $\leq p_i(t)$ **then**
  2:     **if** $p(d_{i,s}) > p_{th}$ **then**
  3:         be_Tentative_Leader $\leftarrow$ TRUE
  4:         Compete_Msg ($RID$, $NID$, $E_{total}(n_i)$)
  5:     **end if**
  6: **end if**
  7: On receiving a COMPETE_MSG from node $n_j$
  8: **if** $RID_j = RID_i$ **then**
  9:     $S_{ni} \leftarrow$ ($n_j$: $n_j$ is a tentative leader)
 10: **end if**
 11: **if** $S_{ni} \neq \emptyset$ **then**
 12:     **if** $E_{total}(n_i) < E_{total}(n_j)$, $\forall n_j \in S_{ni}$ **then**
 13:         be_Final_Leader $\leftarrow$ TRUE
 14:         Leader_Msg($RID$, $NID$, $E_{total}(n_i)$, $d_{i,s}$, $p(d_{i,s})$)
 15:     **else**
 16:         Quit_Msg($RID$, $NID$)
 17:     **end if**
 18: **end if**

**III. Finalize**

  1: **if** be_Final_Leader of node $n_k =$ TRUE **then**
  2:     **if** $d_{i,s} > d_{k,s}$ and $p(d_{i,k}) \cdot p(d_{k,s}) > p(d_{i,s})$ **then**
  3:         node $n_i$ chooses cooperative commun.
  4:     **else**
  5:         node $n_i$ chooses direct commun.
  6:     **end if**
  7: **end if**
  8: **if** be_Final_Leader = FALSE **then**
  9:     return and initialize
 10: **end if**

---

location, initial energy, and residual energy. Then, it contends for a tentative leader with the probability $p_i(t)$ at time $t$, defined as:

$$p_i(t) = \frac{E_i(t)}{E_0}, \qquad (2.14)$$

where $E_i(t)$ is the residual energy and $E_0$ is the initial energy. Note that $p_i(t)$ decreases as the energy is diminished gradually. Thus, to reduce the probability of no tentative leaders and guarantee the network reliability, we add two constraint conditions on $p_i(t)$ and the probability $p(d_{i,s})$ of reliable communication between node $n_i$ and the sink $s$, respectively. Definitely, $p_i(t) > p_{min}$ and $p(d_{i,s}) > p_{th}$, where $p_{min}$ (e.g., $1/N$) and $p_{th}$ are the two thresholds.

Once the expected tentative leaders are elected, they will firstly compute $E_{total}$ by assuming it is the leader and broadcast a COMPETE_MSG message including its *RID*, *NID*, and $E_{total}(n_i)$ to compete the final leader. In order to select the optimal final leader, each tentative leader also maintains a set $S_{ni}$ of its competitors in the same region and compares its total energy consumption $E_{total}$ with its competitors. If $n_i$ finds its $E_{total}$ the lowest, it will successfully be the final leader and broadcast a LEADER_MSG message including its *RID*, *NID*, $E_{total}(n_i)$, $d_{i,s}$, and $p(d_{i,s})$. Otherwise, it will give up the competition immediately and inform other nodes by a QUIT_MSG message.

Finally, if node $n_k$ becomes the final leader, the normal nodes will choose the communication mode according to the reliable and energy-efficient communication strategy. Nevertheless, if there doesn't exist the final leader, it will return to the initialization and reselect the leader.

The leader election process in REELE is message driven, thus we discuss its message exchange complexity below.

**Lemma 2.2** *REELE algorithm has a worst-case message exchange complexity of $O(I)$ in the network, where $I$ is the number of nodes.*

*Proof* During the execution of REELE, there are at most $I \cdot p_i(t)$ tentative leaders who broadcast the COMPETE_MSG per round. Then, each of them either broadcasts a LEADER_MSG to act as the final leader or a QUIT_MSG to be a normal node. For only one final leader is elected in one region, there will be $M$ LEADER_MSGs and $(I \cdot p_i(t) - M)$ QUIT_MSGs are transmitted. After the final leader has been elected, each normal node will send a short control message to the leader to confirm their communication modes. Thus, the messages add up to $2Ip_i(t) + (I - M)$ per round. Since $p_i(t) < 1$, the total asymptotic order of the control overhead is $O(I)$. □

*Remark* The number of nodes in a WBSN is extremely limited for the network characteristics. Consequently, Lemma 2.2 verifies the message overhead of Algorithm 2 is very small.

### 2.5.5 Performance Evaluation

In order to evaluate the performance of REELE, we further compare it with LEACH-A and HEED-A. Without loss of generality, we use the same simulation setting shown in Table 2.2 and the same sensor deployment described in Fig. 2.3 to assess the performance of REELE in terms of network lifetime, the average residual energy, and energy efficiency. Moreover, to justify the improvement in the reliability of REELE, the reliability of each node is investigated as well.

Figure 2.10 illustrates the network lifetime as the initial energy varies. It is shown that REELE algorithm dramatically improves the lifetime over LEACH-A and HEED-A. In REELE, only the node of the more residual energy and less total

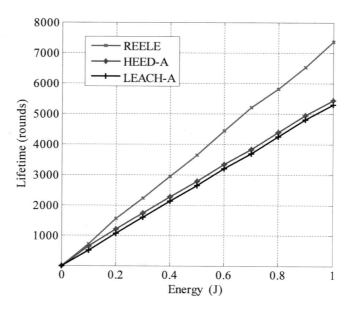

**Fig. 2.10** The network lifetime over initial energy

energy consumption is elected as the leader so that it not only balances the burden of the leader but also reduces the total energy depletion. Differently, LEACH-A requires each node taking its turn to be the leader, while HEED-A only considers residual energy as main criterion to elect the leader.

We now evaluate average residual energy and energy efficiency defined as the ratio of total energy consumption to total received bits. Figures 2.11 and 2.12 manifest that REELE achieves the most residual energy and the lowest energy efficiency. Note that the lower the energy efficiency is, the less energy is expended by transmitting per bit information.

Both LEACH-A and HEED-A overlook the case that a far node also can win as the leader. In this case, it will dissipate more considerable energy to transmit the packets to the sink over a longer distance, which leads to the vast decrease of the residual energy. Thoughtfully, the constraints both on the competitive probability and reliability are used in REELE, dropping the probability of a far node to be the leader. Moreover, the proposed reliable and energy-efficient communication strategy relieves the burden of the leader and far nodes. Consequently, it can achieve more residual energy.

The definition of the energy efficiency implies that under the same amount of the traffic per round, the less energy cost is, the lower energy efficiency can be achieved. Different from LEACH-A and HEED-A, the normal nodes in REELE choose the effective communication mode for themselves according to the reliable and energy-efficient communication strategy. A quantitative comparison can be made from

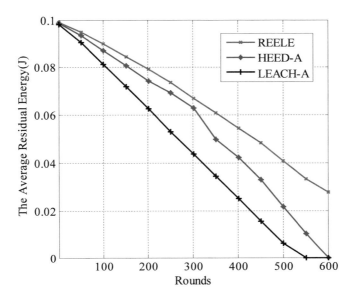

**Fig. 2.11**  The average residual energy over time

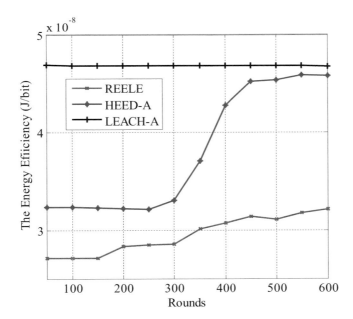

**Fig. 2.12**  The energy efficiency over time

Fig. 2.12 that REELE outperforms LEACH-A and HEED-A over $-42.2\%$ and $-31.6\%$ in energy efficiency, respectively.

In addition, we also draw another interesting observation from Fig. 2.12. The energy efficiency of LEACH-A is always stable, while it goes up rapidly after the time is greater than a certain value in HEED-A. This can be interpreted as follows. In LEACH-A, all nodes play a role as the leader for the same times, so the average energy consumption per bit is almost the same. However, HEED-A primarily considers the residual energy of the nodes, thus a closer node contends for the leader with a bigger probability at the start, while the probability of a farther node to become the leader raises as the residual energy decreases gradually over time, resulting in the increase of energy efficiency.

Figure 2.13 compares the amount of energy spent by the leader per round in three algorithms. To show the results clearly, we present the results on LEACH-A and HEED-A in Fig. 2.13b on a small scale. From Fig. 2.13a, we can see that the energy consumption by the leader per round in REELE is rather less than that in HEED-A and LEACH-A. The reason is twofold. Firstly, the burden of the leader is relieved by using the novel communication strategy in REELE. Secondly, the node with the lowest total energy consumption is elected as the leader.

In addition, a similar observation to that made for energy efficiency in Fig. 2.12 can be made from Fig. 2.13b that the energy consumption of the leader in LEACH-A fluctuates regularly and in HEED-A it keeps low at the beginning and its expected value increase over time.

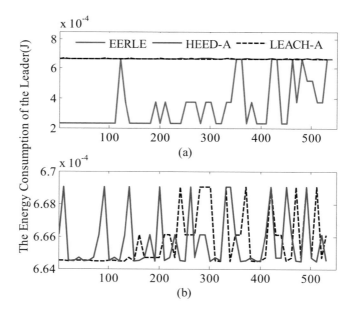

**Fig. 2.13** Energy consumption of leader. (**a, b**) Rounds

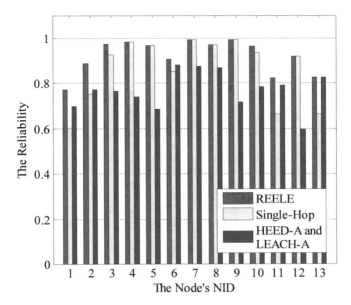

**Fig. 2.14**  The reliability of each node

In order to evaluate the network reliability, in Fig. 2.14 we show the reliability of each node in REELE. Compared with the single hop communication, the use of the reliable and energy-efficient communication strategy in REELE allows a remarkable performance enhancement for the far nodes as well as a good performance guarantee for the close nodes. However, in HEED-A and LEACH-A, the reliability of the close nodes is deteriorated substantially although that of the far nodes is improved slightly.

## 2.6  Conclusion

In this chapter, a set of two novel energy-efficient leader election mechanisms for prolonging the network lifetime are presented in WBSNs. Firstly, a hybrid communication mode is developed such that the burden of the leader and the far node is relieved. Correspondingly, we design a distributed leader election algorithm which comprehensively considers both the residual energy and the location of the node, called EELE. Secondly, we proceed to proposing a reliable and energy-efficient leader election scheme, called REELE, in which we jointly consider the impact of the reliability, the residual energy, and the total energy consumption of a region. Then, the theoretical analysis proves that the overhead of EELE and REELE algorithms is small. Finally, simulation results show that EELE and REELE mechanisms could dramatically reduce the energy consumption, clearly prolong the network lifetime, and extensively increase the network throughput and reliability, respectively.

# References

1. W.B. Heinzelman, A.P. Chandrakasan, H. Balakrishnan, An application-specific protocol architecture for wireless microsensor networks. IEEE Trans. Wirel. Commun. **1**(4), 660–670 (2002)
2. O. Younis, S. Fahmy, HEED: a hybrid, energy-efficient, distributed clustering approach for ad hoc sensor networks. IEEE Trans. Mob. Comput. **3**(4), 366–379 (2004)
3. A. Fort, J. Ryckaert, C. Desset, P. De Doncker, P. Wambacq, L. Van Biesen, Ultra-wideband channel model for communication around the human body. IEEE J. Sel. Areas Commun. **24**(4), 927–933 (2006)
4. R. D'Errico, R. Rosini, M. Maman, A performance evaluation of cooperative schemes for on-body area networks based on measured time-variant channels, in *2011 IEEE International Conference on Communications (ICC)* (IEEE, Piscataway, 2011), pp. 1–5
5. I.S. Association et al., IEEE standard for local and metropolitan area networks-part 15.6: wireless body area networks. IEEE Stand. Inf. Technol. **802**(6), 1–271 (2012)
6. A.A. Abbasi, M. Younis, A survey on clustering algorithms for wireless sensor networks. Comput. Commun. **30**(14), 2826–2841 (2007)
7. O. Boyinbode, H. Le, M. Takizawa, A survey on clustering algorithms for wireless sensor networks. Int. J. Space-Based Situat. Comput. **1**(2–3), 130–136 (2011)
8. R.S. Randriatsiferana, R. Lorion, F. Alicalapa, F. Harivelo, Energy-efficient clustering algorithm based on energy variance for wireless sensor networks, in *2013 International Conference on Smart Communications in Network Technologies (SaCoNeT)*, vol. 1 (IEEE, Piscataway, 2013), pp. 1–5
9. D. Kumar, Performance analysis of energy efficient clustering protocols for maximising lifetime of wireless sensor networks. IET Wireless Sens. Syst. **4**(1), 9–16 (2014)
10. J. Ding, E. Dutkiewicz, X. Huang, G. Fang, Energy-efficient cooperative relay selection for UWB based body area networks, in *2013 IEEE International Conference on Ultra-Wideband (ICUWB)* (IEEE, Piscataway, 2013), pp. 97–102
11. X. Huang, H. Shan, X. Shen, On energy efficiency of cooperative communications in wireless body area network, in *2011 IEEE Wireless Communications and Networking Conference* (IEEE, Piscataway, 2011), pp. 1097–1101
12. E. Reusens, W. Joseph, B. Latré, B. Braem, G. Vermeeren, E. Tanghe, L. Martens, I. Moerman, C. Blondia, Characterization of on-body communication channel and energy efficient topology design for wireless body area networks. IEEE Trans. Inf. Technol. Biomed. **13**(6), 933–945 (2009)

# Chapter 3
# MAC Protocol for Duty-Cycling WBSNs with Concurrent Traffic

**Chapter Roadmap** The rest of this chapter is organized as follows: Section 3.1 explains the motivation of studying MAC protocol and summarizes the contributions. Section 3.2 gives a brief overview of related work in duty-cycling MAC protocols. In Sects. 3.3 and 3.4, we present the system model and introduce the IEEE 802.15.6 CSMA/CA mechanism, respectively. In Sect. 3.5, we detail C-MAC protocol and then develop the theoretical analysis of delay and energy consumption of C-MAC in Sects. 3.6 and 3.7. We evaluate the performance of C-MAC in Sect. 3.8. Finally, we conclude the chapter in Sect. 3.9.

## 3.1 Introduction

### 3.1.1 Context and Motivation

One major application of WBSNs is health care monitoring, where a number of patients can be observed, diagnosed, prescribed remotely as described in Chap. 1. Thus, WBSNs have emerged as a promising alternative to traditional wired network systems for medical environment with significant impact on the rehabilitation and improved patients' quality of life [1]. Specifically, WBSNs can be applied to different scenarios such as monitoring of an individual patient from home, monitoring of few patients from intensive care units (ICU), and monitoring of many patients from hospital wards [2].

Generally, the energy consumption and latency are two important design constraints along with the miniature size of the sensor nodes. Specifically, the energy is consumed mostly for idle listening, collision, and overhearing besides transceiving packets [3]. In idle listening, a node keeps its radio on to listen to an idle channel for receiving possible packets even though no packets have been sent. The collision happens when more than one senders communicate with the same destination

© Springer Nature Switzerland AG 2020
R. Zhang and J. Yu, *Energy-Efficient Algorithms and Protocols for Wireless Body Sensor Networks*, https://doi.org/10.1007/978-3-030-28580-7_3

simultaneously, resulting in corrupted, discarded, or retransmitted events. The overhearing problem occurs when a node receives a packet not originally for it. To cut down the energy waste and prolong the lifetime of sensor nodes, in recent years, many energy-efficient MAC protocols [4] have been designed from the perspective of reducing idle listening, collision, and overhearing.

Moreover, duty-cycling technique is employed in most of MAC protocols to conserve energy by periodically switching between active and sleep states. As introduced in Sect. 3.2, there exist many synchronous and asynchronous duty-cycling MAC protocols for WSNs. However, they are not appropriate to be applied to WBSNs directly in some application scenarios.

Typically in WBSNs, physiological data of various parts of the body are transmitted over the network. Different nodes connected inside or on the body have great variation in terms of data rate. For example, in an ICU room for patient, continuous monitoring of ECG, oxygen, body temperature, and blood pressure could be required. Especially, a WBSN could often experience bursty or concurrent traffic load, when the patient's condition varies, where multiple sensors will send their reports to the sink concurrently, boosting the convergecast traffic load and increasing the channel contention among multiple active sensors which leads to severe collisions. In this case, the existing MAC protocols will become less efficient in delay and energy efficiency, because this concurrent traffic in the latency-sensitive applications is ignored in their design. Therefore, it is necessary to design an energy-efficient MAC protocol for duty-cycling WBSNs.

## 3.1.2  Summary of Contributions

Motivated by the observations, in this chapter we present an asynchronous duty-cycling MAC protocol for concurrent traffic load, called C-MAC. C-MAC attempts to avoid collisions of concurrent flows to reduce the packet transmission delay and conserve energy, i.e., ensuring that multiple detected physiological parameters can accurately and timely be received by the sink to the maximum extent such that the actuator can make the accurate diagnoses in the medical applications.

Definitely, C-MAC exploits the receiver-initiated approach, which removes the pressure on the battery from the sensor nodes to the sink, considering the characteristics of WBSNs that the sink is more powerful than sensor nodes, such as the operability of recharge or replacement.

Moreover, differing from the existing MAC protocols, C-MAC focuses on handling collisions, idle listening, and overhearing problems in medical applications with the concurrent traffic load. Therefore, the main contributions of this chapter are articulated as follows:

- Firstly, we propose a two-phase asynchronous duty-cycling MAC protocol, called C-MAC. In the first phase, the IEEE 802.15.6 CSMA/CA mechanism is employed to avoid collisions among the control messages exchanges. Moreover, an ordering-based communication algorithm is designed to sequence data packet transmissions. In the second phase, we introduce standby mode (SBM) so that nodes can switch to this mode, reducing the idle listening and overhearing among data transmissions.

- Secondly, we explicitly derive the mathematical formulas of the random delay and the normalized energy consumption for C-MAC. Subsequently, we validate the correctness of theoretical analysis in terms of the mean and variance by simulation and numerical results.
- Finally, we conduct extensive simulation to evaluate the performance of C-MAC by comparing with RI-MAC and A-MAC. The simulation results demonstrate that C-MAC significantly conserves energy and reduces the transmission delay, especially under concurrent traffic.

To the best of our knowledge, we believe that this is the first effort to address the concurrent traffic in the medical applications of WBSNs by designing an IEEE 802.15.6 CSMA/CA and ordering-based receiver-initiated asynchronous duty-cycling MAC protocol.

## 3.2  Related Work

Generally, the energy is consumed mostly for idle listening, collision, and overhearing for nodes in WBSNs [5]. Specifically, in idle listening, a node keeps its radio on to listen to an idle channel for receiving possible packets even though no packets have been sent. The collision happens when more than one senders communicate with the same destination simultaneously, resulting in corrupted, discarded, or retransmitted events. The overhearing problem occurs when a node receives a packet not originally for it. A well-designed MAC protocol can effectively prolong the overall network lifetime [6]. Thus, in order to reduce the energy waste and prolong the lifetime of sensor nodes, in recent years, many energy-efficient MAC protocols [4] have been designed from the perspective of reducing idle listening, collision, and overhearing, in which the duty-cycling MAC protocols have attracted a lot of attention [7].

By duty cycling, each node periodically turns on/off its radio to alternate between active and sleep states. Based on the synchronization requirement, the existing duty-cycling MAC protocols can be roughly categorized into two types: *synchronous* and *asynchronous*.

In synchronous protocols such as T-MAC [8], RMAC [9], Mix-MAC [10], iA-MAC [11], RTS-MAC [12], and MRPM [13], neighbor nodes exchange control message to schedule transmissions, which greatly reduces idle listening, but periodic time synchronization incurs much extra overhead. In addition, it is inefficient in handling variable rate traffic to use fixed duty cycle period.

In contrast, asynchronous duty-cycling protocols that do not require synchronization allow nodes to have their individual duty cycles. Depending on which end of a communication link initiates a transfer, the asynchronous protocols may be further classified as either *sender-initiated* or *receiver-initiated*, which are discussed detailed as follows.

**Sender-Initiated Protocols** B-MAC [14] and X-MAC [15] are primary sender-initiated asynchronous duty-cycling protocols. In B-MAC, the authors exploit low power listening (LPL) mechanism, in which, before data transmission, the sender with pending packets first transmits a preamble lasting at least as long as the sleep period of the receiver. When the receiver wakes up and detects the preamble, it will remain awake to receive the subsequent packets. This approach can achieve high energy efficiency under light traffic loads. The efficiency of B-MAC, however, degrades as the traffic loads increase due to the long preamble transmission.

X-MAC [15] attempts to resolve this problem by dividing the long preamble into a series of short preambles embedded with the address of the target node such that all other nodes except the intended receiver deactivate themselves immediately. Consequently, X-MAC can effectively avoid overhearing and save energy. The channel utilization, however, is still low in X-MAC for the consecutive preambles.

Subsequently, a prediction-based mechanism is proposed in WiseMAC [16], where the sender can first predict the next wake-up time of the receiver by learning its duty cycle and send a shortened preamble just before the receiver wakes up. WiseMAC thus can improve the channel utilization and save energy. But hidden terminal problem and persistent collisions will often happen once the nodes choose the approximately same wake-up time, because the nodes maintain the same fixed duty cycle period over time.

Due to the drawbacks of sender-initiated protocols, researchers turn their attention to receiver-initiated approach which can handle hidden terminal problem, achieve low power probing, support low duty cycles and high data rate [17].

**Receiver-Initiated Protocols** In RI-MAC [18], the receiver immediately broadcasts a beacon after its wakeup, announcing that it is awake and ready to receive packets. Upon the beacon reception, the sender transmits its packet immediately. If there are multiple active senders, a collision will happen and be detected. Then, the receiver sends another beacon with increased backoff window value to request the senders to do a backoff before their next transmission attempts in order to avoid repeated collisions. However, the efficiency of RI-MAC degrades under the concurrent traffic loads and the overhearing cannot be resolved in RI-MAC.

Differing from RI-MAC, A-MAC [19] requires the sender to send back an auto-ACK after receiving the preamble, which helps the sink determine whether a packet is pending. Then, the sender transmits a packet after a short and random delay. Whereas once the ACKs or packets collide, the receiver transmits another probe with an explicit contention window to request the senders to retransmit packets. Once a node wins the other nodes keep backoff status to avoid collisions. However, the efficiency of A-MAC degrades under the concurrent traffic load as the collision avoidance has not been considered in advance.

Armed with a novel on-demand prediction error correction mechanism, PW-MAC [20] effectively minimizes the energy consumption of sensor nodes by enabling senders to predict receiver wake-up time. Moreover, an efficient prediction-based retransmission mechanism is designed in PW-MAC to achieve high energy efficiency. When a node recognizes the failure of its transmission, it switches to sleeping state and wakes up at the next predicted receiver wake-up time to retransmit the packet, thereby minimizing the energy consumption spending on waiting for the receiver. However, for the sake of accurate prediction, PW-MAC requests the nodes to persistently learn and update the prediction state of its neighbors, which needs more memory and increases message overhead.

Subsequently, a traffic-aware dynamic MAC (TAD-MAC) protocol is proposed in [21] differing the topologies constructed by on-body sensors and in-body sensors. In TAD-MAC, each node maintains a traffic status register bank which contains the traffic statistics of all its neighbor nodes to update its wake-up interval dynamically with due account of the amount of traffic. Similar with PW-MAC, TAD-MAC also results in more memory and heavy message overhead.

Recently, a receiver-centric MAC (RC-MAC) protocol is presented in [22] to handle bursty traffic triggered by the event. RC-MAC takes advantage of the data gathering tree structure and multi-channel technique to assist scheduling of medium access to improve the throughput in two phases. First, a receiver is able to coordinate the medium access of several senders so as to reduce collisions and achieve high throughput on a data gathering tree. Second different sender–receiver pairs can communicate in different channels, thus the throughput can be further improved by allowing the parallel data gathering. However, the overhead and energy consumption are very heavy as each node needs to periodically update the beacon offset of all its neighbors to obtain link information in RC-MAC.

It is worth noticing that all the aforementioned MAC protocols cannot be directly applied in WBSNs with bursty or concurrent traffic. The main reason is that the collision probability is very high when multiple nodes concurrently communicate with the same destination; however, the collision avoidance has not been considered in advance in prior protocols, which can result in the persistent collisions among nodes and increase the energy consumption and the transmission delay. Therefore, it is necessary to design a duty-cycling MAC protocol for WBSNs to handle the collisions, idle listening, and overhearing problems in medical applications with concurrent traffic loads. Table 3.1 compares the existing asynchronous duty-cycling MAC protocols.

## 3.3 System Model

Duty cycling, as an effective energy saving technique, is employed in most of the sensor networks. However, it will lead to significant latency in packet delivery, since the senders have to wait until the receiver wakes up to transmit packets. Despite some existing protocols attempt to mitigate the additional latency, they only work

**Table 3.1** Comparison of the duty-cycling MAC protocols

| Protocols | Initiated end | Collision | Overhead | Bursty traffic |
|-----------|---------------|-----------|----------|----------------|
| B-MAC | Sender | Very high | Low | No |
| X-MAC | Sender | High | Low | No |
| WiseMAC | Sender | High | Very high | No |
| RI-MAC | Receiver | Low | High | No |
| A-MAC | Receiver | Low | Very high | No |
| PW-MAC | Receiver | Low | Very high | No |
| TAD-MAC | Receiver | Low | Very high | No |
| RC-MAC | Receiver | Very low | Very high | Yes |
| C-MAC | Receiver | Very rare | Low | Yes |

effectively under light traffic load. However, a WBSN could often experience bursty or concurrent traffic, especially in health monitoring applications. When the status of a patient changes, multiple sensors will send their reports to the sink concurrently, boosting the convergecast traffic load and increasing the channel contention among multiple active sensors which leads to severe collisions. In this case, to accurately detect the patient's health condition, the physician needs the real-time data from sensors and comprehensively analyzes the data. Therefore, it is essential to design a MAC protocol to accommodate this concurrent traffic in medical applications.

In these scenarios, we consider a popular single-hop star WBSN network of a sink and multiple sensor nodes where the sink plays the role of the receiver. A reasonable assumption that the collision is the only cause of packet transmission failure under perfect channel condition is adopted.

In duty-cycling protocols, the sink and each node alternatively stay in two major states based on their individual schedule, i.e.,

- Active state: The sink and the node turn on their radio and stay awake for normal operations, such as transmitting or receiving packets.
- Sleep state: The sink and the node completely shut down to conserve energy.

Moreover, in order to avoid idle listening and overhearing and reduce energy consumption for the nodes during data packet transmission, inspired by Tuck [23], Atmel Corporation [24], we further introduce SBM, i.e.,

- Standby mode: All the operations of the node are stopped except the system clock, thus the node can save energy and also promptly switch to active state to transmit packets.

Figure 3.1 illustrates the transition relationship among these states. Note that only the node can switch between the active state and the SBM.

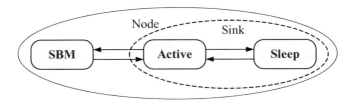

**Fig. 3.1** State transition relationship

## 3.4   Overview of IEEE 802.15.6 CSMA/CA Protocol

Here, we briefly introduce the CSMA/CA mechanism specified in IEEE 802.15.6 standard [25], which will be used in the follow-up design and analysis of C-MAC protocol.

To meet the MAC needs of low-power and short-range WBSNs, the CSMA/CA mechanism has been developed and employed in IEEE 802.15.6 standard. In this mechanism, a node should maintain three variables for each transmission attempt: $NB$, $CW$, and $BC$, where $NB$ is the number of backoff times, $CW$ is the value of contention window, and $BC$ is the backoff counter. A formal description of IEEE 802.15.6 CSMA/CA mechanism is shown in Algorithm 1 for an arbitrary node.

---

**Algorithm 1** IEEE 802.15.6 CSMA/CA mechanism

---

**Require:** $CW_{min}, CW_{max}, NB$
 1: **Initialisation:** $BC = random\,(1, CW)$
 2: $NB{+}{+}$
 3: **if** *channel is idle* **then**
 4:     $BC{-}{-}$
 5:     **if** $BC{=}{=}0$ **then**
 6:         Transmit data
 7:         **if** $n_i$ failed **then**
 8:             **if** $NB$ is even **then**
 9:                 Double $CW$
10:                 **if** $CW > CW_{max}$ **then**
11:                     $CW = CW_{max}$
12:                 **end if**
13:             **else**
14:                 $CW$ is unchanged
15:             **end if**
16:         **end if**
17:     **end if**
18: **else**
19:     Lock $BC$ until channel is idle
20: **end if**

---

First, after sensing the channel is idle for a short interframe spacing (SIFS) time interval for an arbitrary node $n_i$, it initializes its $BC$ to a random integer uniformly distributed over the interval $[1, CW]$, where $CW \in (CW_{min}, CW_{max})$. The values of $CW_{min}$ and $CW_{max}$ depend on the priority of a user. Subsequently, the node decreases $BC$ by one for each idle CSMA/CA slot. Otherwise, the node locks the $BC$ until the channel is idle again. Once the $BC$ reaches zero and the channel is idle, the node can send its packet. Meanwhile, the number of $NB$ increases by one for each access attempt. If the contention fails, $CW$ is doubled for even number of failures, and remains unchanged for odd number of failures. If the doubling $CW$ exceeds the $CW_{max}$, the node sets the $CW$ to $CW_{max}$. Then, the node will select a new $BC$ over new $[1, CW]$ and repeat the backoff procedure in the following slots until the packet is transmitted successfully or it reaches the maximum number of backoff $NB_{max}$. Note that the initial $CW$ is generally set to $CW_{min}$.

## 3.5  C-MAC Description

### 3.5.1  Overview of C-MAC

The C-MAC consists of two phases: the *control message exchange* phase and the *data packet transmission* phase. Figure 3.2 illustrates an example of the operation of C-MAC.

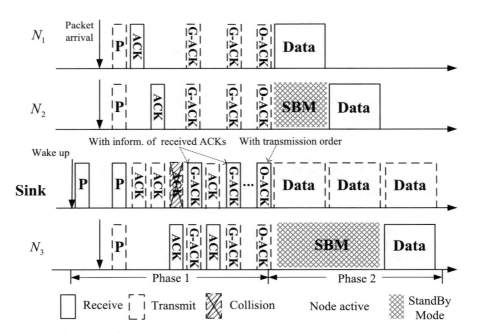

**Fig. 3.2**  Illustration of C-MAC

**Phase 1-Control Message Exchange**  After turning on its radio, the sink broadcasts a preamble, announcing that it is awake and ready to receive packets. Then the sink will wait for the feedback from nodes. For the nodes with pending packets, they stay silent to wait for the preamble from the sink. Upon receiving a preamble, the active nodes will respond ACKs following the IEEE 802.15.6 CSMA/CA mechanism. Once receiving ACKs, the sink realizes the success of its preamble transmission, while instead of replying with an I-ACK (Immediate-ACK) it waits for all probable ACKs from the other active nodes triggered by the same event and sends a G-ACK (Group-ACK) with the information of received ACKs after a timeout. Otherwise, the sink will transmit another preamble with random backoff until it receives ACKs successfully or it reaches the maximum number of the preambles $N_p$. Note that the G-ACK's role is two-fold: On the one hand, it reports the correct receipt of ACKs of which nodes, and it informs the nodes whose ACKs were collided to resend their ACKs subsequently, on the other hand. After the reception of G-ACK, each node firstly checks whether its ACK has been received successfully. If so, the node will wait for O-ACK (Organized-ACK); otherwise, it will retransmit its ACK and wait for G-ACK. If there is no incoming ACK in a timeout after transmitting a G-ACK, the sink regards itself having received all ACKs successfully and executes the ordering-based communication algorithm subsequently described in Algorithm 2 to sequence all nodes' data packet transmissions and broadcasts an O-ACK with nodes' communication order. Specifically, the O-ACK can acknowledge all ACKs and also notice the start of the data packet transmission phase. If there is not any feedback after the $N_p$-th preamble transmission, the sink realizes that there is no incoming packet and switches to sleep state.

**Phase 2-Data Packet Transmission**  Once receiving O-ACK, each node will compute its accurate transmission time according to its order. Thus, it can decide to remain active to transmit packet or switch to the SBM until just before its due transmission time. If the node does not find its communication order in O-ACK, it will sleep immediately. Once the O-ACK is lost, the sink will retransmit until O-ACK is successful or it reaches the maximum transmission times $N_o$. Under the concurrent traffic load, C-MAC significantly reduces the transmission delay resulted from persistent collisions by combining IEEE 802.15.6 CSMA/CA and ordering-based communication algorithm. Moreover, the design of G-ACK and O-ACK enables that the sink can receive concurrent packets as many as possible in one duty cycle period and resolve the early sleep problem [26] that the sink goes to sleep when some other active nodes still have packets to transmit. Furthermore, C-MAC dramatically reduces the energy consumption incurred by the idle listening and overhearing by the design of SBM.

### 3.5.2  Ordering-Based Communication Algorithm

We here elaborate the ordering-based communication algorithm executed by the sink.

As shown in Algorithm 2, there are four inputs, namely the timeout duration $T_{out}$, the maximum number of preambles $N_p$, the maximum number of G-ACKs $N_a$, and the maximum number of O-ACKs $N_o$. With these inputs, the sink initializes the following parameters: two time counters $C_s$ and $C_d$, the current number of preambles $k_p$, the current number of G-ACKs $k_a$ and the current number of O-ACKs $k_o$, and the set of received ACKs $S_{ack}$ and the set of received data packets $S_{data}$. Then, the sink receives probable ACKs and adds them to the set $S_{ack}$ in a $T_{out}$ as lines 2–4. If $S_{ack}$ is not empty, the sink sends back a G-ACK, resets the counter $C_s$, and repeats the procedures 2–4 to further receive ACKs from active nodes. If there is no incoming ACK when $T_{out}$ expires, the sink then sequences the data

---

**Algorithm 2** Ordering-based communication algorithm

**Require:** $T_{out}, N_p, N_a, N_o$.
  1: **Initialization:** counters $C_s = 0, C_d = 0$, and $k_p, k_a, k_o, S_{ack} = \emptyset, S_{data} = \emptyset$.
  2: **while** $C_s < T_{out}$ **do**
  3:    Receive $ACK$, $S_{ack} = S_{ack} \cup ACK$
  4: **end while**
  5: **if** $|S_{ack}| \geq 1$ **then**
  6:    $N_{ack} = |S_{ack}|$
  7:    **if** $k_a < N_a$ **then**
  8:       Send G-ACK, $k_a$++
  9:       reset $C_s = 0$ and repeat 2–4
 10:       **if** $|S_{ack}| > N_{ack}$ **then**
 11:          Repeat 6–9
 12:       **else**
 13:          Sequence the data packet transmission
 14:          Send O-ACK
 15:          **while** $C_d < T_{SIFS} + T_{data}$ **do**
 16:             Receive $DATA$, $S_{data} = S_{data} \cup DATA$
 17:          **end while**
 18:          **if** $|S_{data}|==0$ **then**
 19:             $k_o$++
 20:             **if** $k_o < N_o$ **then**
 21:                Repeat 14–17
 22:             **else**
 23:                Turn off the radio
 24:             **end if**
 25:          **else**
 26:             Continue to receive data packets
 27:          **end if**
 28:       **end if**
 29:    **else**
 30:       Execute 14–28
 31:    **end if**
 32: **else if** $k_p < N_p$ **then**
 33:    Send another preamble, $k_p$++
 34:    Execute 1–31
 35: **else**
 36:    Turn off the radio
 37: **end if**

packet transmissions for all active nodes following some given sorting algorithm and sends an O-ACK. Subsequently, if the sink does not receive any data packet within $T_{SIFS} + T_{data}$ and $k_o < N_o$, it repeats 14–17. Otherwise, the sink continues to receive packets from the others. If $S_{ack}$ is empty and $k_p$ does not reach to $N_p$, the sink transmits a new preamble in order to receive possible ACKs. Then, the sink returns to the initialization and repeats lines 2–31. If not receiving any ACK after sending $N_p$ preambles, the sink turns off its radio and switches to sleep state.

## 3.6  Delay Analysis

In this section, we explicitly formulate the mathematical expression of the delay $T_d$ which is the duration between the packet arrival at a node and its successful reception by the sink. For deriving $T_d$, we need to calculate the following components:

- $T_1$: random delay spent by the sink to accomplish a successful preamble transmission.
- $T_w$: random delay spent by the node from the instant of packet arrival until a successful reception of preamble.
- $T_o$: random delay spent by the node from the reception of a preamble until the reception of O-ACK.
- $T_c$: random delay spent by the node from the O-ACK reception until the transmission of a packet.

As shown in Fig. 3.3, the delay for an arbitrary node $N_m$ to successfully send a data packet is thus $T_d = T_w + T_o + T_c$. Next, we formally derive these delay components in sequence. Note that Table 3.2 lists the main symbols used in the performance analysis of C-MAC protocol.

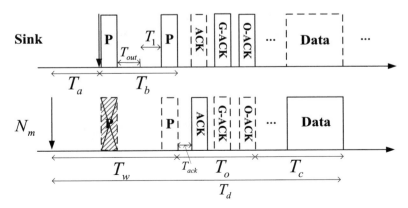

**Fig. 3.3**  An illustration of delay $T_d$

**Table 3.2**  Main symbols

| Symbols | Descriptions |
|---|---|
| $T_{on}$ | Active duration of the sink in one duty-cycling period |
| $T_s$ | Sleep duration of the sink in one duty-cycling period |
| $T_d$ | Transmission delay spent by a node from the instant of packet arrival until its reception successfully by the sink |
| $T_1$ | Random delay spent by the sink before transmitting a preamble |
| $T_w$ | Random delay spent by the node from the instant of waking up until a successful reception of preamble |
| $T_o$ | Random delay spent by the node from the reception of a preamble until the reception of O-ACK |
| $T_c$ | Random delay spent by the node from the O-ACK reception until the transmission of a packet |
| $T_{out}$ | Maximum time that the sink waits for ACKs after having sent a preamble |
| $T_{ack}$ | Random delay spent by the node to send back an ACK to the sink |
| $T_a$ | Random time spent by the node to wait from its wake up to the wake-up instant of the sink as the event $\mathscr{B}$ is true |
| $T_b$ | Time interval from the wake-up moment of the sink until the node succeeds in receiving one preamble as $\mathscr{B}$ is true |
| $T_a'$ | Time interval between the wake-up instants of the sink and nodes given that the event $\mathscr{B}$ is false |
| $T_b'$ | Random delay spent by the sink from its wake-up moment until a successful reception of one preamble as $\mathscr{B}$ is false |
| $T_p$ | Maximum time duration spent by the sink to transmit preambles |
| $T_{SIFS}$ | Short interframe spacing interval |
| $T_{data}$ | Delay to transmit a packet |
| $T_{hr}$ | Delay employed by the hardware platform to process a packet |
| $E_{N_m}$ | Energy consumption spent by $N_m$ to transmit a packet successfully |
| $E_{sink}$ | Energy consumption spent by the sink during its active duration |
| $N_b$ | Maximum number of backoffs of a preamble |
| $N_p$ | Maximum number of preambles that can be sent by the sink |
| $N_a$ | Maximum number of G-ACK that can be sent by the sink |
| $N_o$ | Maximum number of O-ACK that can be sent by the sink |
| $S_b$ | Unit backoff time used by the CSMA/CA algorithm |
| $S_p$ | Preamble packet duration |
| $L_p$ | Payload of one packet in bits |
| $R_s$ | Data rate in bits/s as in IEEE 802.15.6 standard |
| $\alpha$ | Probability of busy channel |
| $\tau$ | Probability of the node attempting to transmit in a random time slot |
| $\lambda$ | Packet arrival rate per node |
| $t_{p,k,j}$ | Random backoff time before the $j$th attempt to transmit a preamble as the event $\mathscr{A}_k$ happens |

(continued)

**Table 3.2**  (continued)

| Symbols | Descriptions |
|---|---|
| $\mathscr{A}_k$ | Event that the channel is busy for $k-1$ times and free at the $k$th time |
| $\mathscr{B}$ | Event that the sink is sleeping when the nodes wake up to transmit packets |
| $\mathscr{C}_k$ | Event that the sink has to send $k$ preambles before being received and the ACK is sent back before timeout |
| $\mathscr{P}_j$ | Event that a preamble or an ACK is lost at time index $j$ due to collisions |
| $\mathscr{D}_k$ | Event that the sink transmits $k$ preambles before expiration of $T_p$ |
| $\mathscr{F}_k$ | Event that an ACK is transmitted successfully before timeout of the sink in case that $\mathscr{D}_k$ is true |
| $\mathscr{N}_k$ | Event that the $k-1$th preamble is sent but the nodes are sleeping |
| $\mathscr{E}_k$ | Event that the $k$th preamble is sent and the nodes have woken up |
| $\mathscr{R}_n$ | Event that the sink has to send $n$ G-ACKs until no ACK is received |
| $\mathscr{Q}_l$ | Event that the $l$th O-ACK is received successfully by the nodes |

### 3.6.1  Modeling of $T_1$

Assume that the mechanism to transmit a preamble for the sink is the same with an ACK message transmission for nodes as specified in IEEE 802.15.6 CSMA/CA in Sect. 3.4. Let $\alpha$ be the probability of busy channel which is approximately independent at each attempt for each node [27]. Let $N_b$ be the maximum number of backoffs of a preamble, i.e., to access the channel the sink can transmit at most $N_b$ preambles.

Let $t_{p,k,j}$ be the random backoff time before the $j$th attempt to transmit a preamble for the case where the channel is busy for $k-1$ times and free at the $k$th time. It follows that $t_{p,k,j}$ has a uniform distribution over the interval $[1, CW_{k,j}] \cdot S_b$, where $S_b$ is a unit backoff time used by the CSMA/CA mechanism. Denote by $\mathscr{A}_k$ the event that the channel is busy for $k-1$ times and free at the $k$th time, and by $\mathscr{A}$ the event that a preamble is transmitted with at maximum $N_b$ backoffs. Thus, random delay $T_1$ spent by the sink before transmitting a preamble within $N_b$ attempts can be expressed as

$$T_1 = \sum_{k=1}^{N_b} \left( \sum_{j=1}^{k} t_{p,k,j} \right) \mathbb{1}_{\mathscr{A}_k | \mathscr{A}} = \sum_{k=1}^{N_b} \Sigma_k \mathbb{1}_{\mathscr{A}_k | \mathscr{A}}, \tag{3.1}$$

where $\mathbb{1}_{(\cdot)}$ is the indicator function ($\mathbb{1}_{(\cdot)} = 1$ if the argument is true, and $\mathbb{1}_{(\cdot)} = 0$ otherwise) and $\Sigma_k = \sum_{j=1}^{k} t_{p,k,j}$ is the random variable describing the time spent for the $k$th random backoff. Note that the primitive backoff for the first preamble first attempt is set to 0, i.e., $t_{p,1,1} = 0$ in this chapter. Consequently, we can obtain the probabilistic characteristics of $T_1$ as stated in the following Lemma 3.1.

**Lemma 3.1** *The mean and variance of $T_1$ are*

$$\mu_{T_1} = \mathbb{E}[T_1] = \sum_{k=1}^{N_b} \mu_{\Sigma_k} \frac{\alpha^{k-1}}{\sum_{j=1}^{N_b} \alpha^{j-1}}, \quad \sigma_{T_1} = \mathbb{E}[T_1 - \mathbb{E}[T_1]]^2 = \sum_{k=1}^{N_b} \sigma_{\Sigma_k}^2 \frac{\alpha^{k-1}}{\sum_{j=1}^{N_b} \alpha^{j-1}},$$

*where $\mathbb{E}[\cdot]$ defines the mean of a random variable and*

$$\mu_{\Sigma_k} = \mathbb{E}[\Sigma_k] = \sum_{j=1}^{k} \mu_{t_{p,k,j}}, \quad \sigma_{\Sigma_k}^2 = \mathbb{E}[\Sigma_k - \mathbb{E}[\Sigma_k]]^2 = \sum_{j=1}^{k} \sigma_{t_{p,k,j}}^2,$$

*where $\mu_{t_{p,k,j}}$ and $\sigma_{t_{p,k,j}}^2$ denote the mean and variance of the random variable $t_{p,k,j}$.*

*Proof* Since $\mathscr{A}_k$ is the event that the channel is busy for $k-1$ times and free at the $k$th time, the probability of this event is $\Pr(\mathscr{A}_k) = \alpha^{k-1}(1-\alpha)$. The probability that the event $\mathscr{A}$ establishes is then derived as

$$\Pr(\mathscr{A}) = \Pr\left(\sum_{j=1}^{N_b} \mathscr{A}_j\right) = \sum_{j=1}^{N_b} \Pr(\mathscr{A}_j),$$

where the equality comes from that the events $\mathscr{A}_j$, $j = 1, \ldots, N_b$ are mutually exclusive. It thus also holds that

$$\Pr(\mathscr{A}_k \mid \mathscr{A}) = \frac{\Pr(\mathscr{A}_k \sum_{j=1}^{N_b} \mathscr{A}_j)}{\Pr(\mathscr{A})} = \frac{\Pr(\mathscr{A}_k)}{\sum_{j=1}^{N_b} \Pr(\mathscr{A}_j)} = \frac{\alpha^{k-1}}{\sum_{j=1}^{N_b} \alpha^{j-1}}.$$

Since $\Sigma_k$ is the sum of independent uniformly distributed random variables, its mean can be given by $\mu_{\Sigma_k} = \mathbb{E}[\Sigma_k] = \sum_{j=1}^{k} \mu_{t_{p,k,j}}$, where $\mu_{t_{p,k,j}} = (CW_{k,j} - 1)S_b/2$ [27], and its variance thus equals the sum of the variance of $t_{p,k,j}$, i.e., $\sigma_{\Sigma_k}^2 = \mathbb{E}[\Sigma_k - \mathbb{E}[\Sigma_k]]^2 = \sum_{j=1}^{k} \sigma_{t_{p,k,j}}^2$, where $\sigma_{t_{p,k,j}}^2 = (CW_{k,j} - 1)^2 S_b^2/12$. By using $\mu_{\Sigma_k}$ and $\sigma_{\Sigma_k}^2$ and the properties of the expectation operator, Lemma 3.1 follows.                                                                                   □

*Remark* Since $T_1$ is the weighted sum of uniform random variables with different mean and variance, no closed-form expression is available for the probability mass function. However, a Gaussian distribution can approximate the probability mass function of $T_1$.

In addition, since the ACK message is transmitted with the same backoff mechanism of the preamble, the random delay $T_{ack}$ spent by one node to send back successfully an ACK message to the sink can be approximated by a Gaussian distribution with mean and variance given as

$$\mu_{T_{ack}} = \sum_{k=1}^{N_b} \mu_{\Sigma_k} \frac{\alpha^{k-1}}{\sum_{k=1}^{N_b} \alpha^{k-1}}, \quad \sigma_{T_{ack}}^2 = \sum_{k=1}^{N_b} \sigma_{\Sigma_k}^2 \frac{\alpha^{k-1}}{\sum_{k=1}^{N_b} \alpha^{k-1}}.$$

## 3.6.2 Modeling of $T_w$

In this subsection we model $T_w$ that the random delay between the wake-up moment of a node and the reception moment of a successful preamble followed by an ACK message which is sent back successfully to the sink before timeout. Due to the implementation of asynchronous duty-cycling protocol, we proceed to derive $T_w$ in the following two cases:

$$T_w = \begin{cases} T_a + T_b, & \text{Case 1} : \text{Sink is sleeping,} \\ T_b' - T_a', & \text{Case 2} : \text{Sink is awake.} \end{cases} \tag{3.2}$$

*Case 1* The sink is sleeping when the node wakes up and intends to transmit data packet. The aforementioned Fig. 3.3 shows an illustration for an arbitrary node.

First, denote by $T_a$ the random time for the node to wait from its waking up moment to the instant of the sink waking up. $T_a = 0\mathbb{1}_{\bar{\mathscr{B}}} + T_2\mathbb{1}_{\mathscr{B}}$, where the event $\mathscr{B}$ occurs when the sink is sleeping at the moment that the node has data packet to transmit, and $T_2$ is the random time to wait for the wakeup of the sink given that the event $\mathscr{B}$ is true. Consequently, the probabilities of $\mathscr{B}$ and $\bar{\mathscr{B}}$ are

$$\Pr(\mathscr{B}) = \frac{T_s}{T_{on} + T_s}, \quad \Pr(\bar{\mathscr{B}}) = 1 - \Pr(\mathscr{B}),$$

where $T_s$ and $T_{on}$ are the duration of the sleep and activation of the sink during one duty-cycling period, respectively. As the definition that $\Pr(T_a = 0) = \Pr(\bar{\mathscr{B}})$. Furthermore, since $T_2$ has a uniform distribution in the range $[0, T_s]$, thus the probability of $T_a$ for $0 < T_a \leq T_s$ is given by

$$\Pr(T_a) = \Pr(T_2)\Pr(\mathscr{B}) = \Pr(T_2)\frac{T_s}{T_{on} + T_s}.$$

Therefore, the probability mass function of $T_a$ is

$$\Pr(T_a) = \begin{cases} \frac{1}{T_{on}+T_s} & 0 < T_a \leq T_s, \\ \frac{T_{on}}{T_{on}+T_s} & T_a = 0. \end{cases}$$

We then define $T_b$ as the time interval from the wake-up moment of the sink until one preamble is received successfully by the node given that the event $\mathscr{B}$ is true, as shown in Fig. 3.3. In order to avoid that the sink spends much energy on transmitting preambles as there is no incoming packets for long time, the maximum number of preambles that the sink can transmit is restrained as $N_p$. Furthermore, define $\mathscr{C}_k$ as the event that the sink has to send $k$ preambles before being received and the corresponding ACK is sent back and received before the timeout of the sink. Thus, the random delay of $T_b$ can be formulated as

$$T_b = \sum_{k=1}^{N_p} \left( \sum_{j=1}^{k} T_{1,k,j} + (k-1)T_{out} \right) \mathbb{1}_{\mathscr{C}_k \mid \mathscr{C}}, \tag{3.3}$$

where $T_{1,k,j}$ is the random delay of the transmission of the $j$th preamble when the $k$th preamble with the distribution given in Eq. (3.1) is received successfully by the nodes. $T_{out}$ is defined as the maximum time for the sink to wait for ACKs after having sent a preamble. And $\mathscr{C}$ is the event that the sink receives ACKs within $N_p$ preambles. We next present the probabilistic characteristics of $T_b$ in Lemma 3.2.

**Lemma 3.2** *The mean and variance of $T_b$ are*

$$\mu_{T_b} = \sum_{k=1}^{N_p} \left( k\mu_{T_1} + (k-1)T_{out} \right) \frac{\Pr(\mathscr{C}_k)}{\sum_{j=1}^{N_p} \Pr(\mathscr{C}_j)}, \quad \sigma_{T_b}^2 = \sum_{k=1}^{N_p} \sigma_{T_{b,k}}^2 \frac{\Pr(\mathscr{C}_k)}{\sum_{j=1}^{N_p} \Pr(\mathscr{C}_j)},$$

*where $\sigma_{T_{b,k}}^2$ is the variance of $\sum_{j=1}^{k} T_{1,k,j} + (k-1)T_{out}$, and*

$$\Pr(\mathscr{C}_k) = [\Pr\left( kT_1 + (k-1)T_{out} \leq T_p \right)(1 - \Pr(T_{ack} \leq T_{out}))$$
$$\times \Pr(T_{ack} \leq T_{out})\Pr(\bar{\mathscr{P}}_1)]$$
$$+ [\Pr\left( kT_1 + (k-1)T_{out} \leq T_p \right) \times \Pr(T_{ack} \leq T_{out})^2 \Pr(\mathscr{P}_1)\Pr(\bar{\mathscr{P}}_2)],$$

*where $T_p$ is the maximum time duration to transmit $N_p$ preambles for the sink.*

*Proof* The proof is based on expressing the mean and variance of $T_b$ in terms of $\Pr(\mathscr{C}_k)$. According to the expression of $T_b$ in Eq. (3.3), its mean and variance can be presented as

$$\mu_{T_b} = \sum_{k=1}^{N_p} \left( k\mu_{T_1} + (k-1)T_{out} \right) \Pr(\mathscr{C}_k \mid \mathscr{C}), \quad \sigma_{T_b}^2 = \sum_{k=1}^{N_p} \sigma_{T_{b,k}}^2 \Pr(\mathscr{C}_k \mid \mathscr{C}).$$

Using the fact that the events $\mathscr{C}_j$, $j = 1, \ldots, N_p$ are mutually exclusive, we have

$$\Pr(\mathscr{C}) = \Pr\left( \sum_{k=1}^{N_p} \mathscr{C}_k \right) = \sum_{k=1}^{N_p} \Pr(\mathscr{C}_k),$$

and then

$$\Pr(\mathscr{C}_k \mid \mathscr{C}) = \frac{\Pr\left( \mathscr{C}_k \sum_{j=1}^{N_p} \mathscr{C}_j \right)}{\Pr(\mathscr{C})} = \frac{\Pr(\mathscr{C}_k)}{\sum_{j=1}^{N_p} \Pr(\mathscr{C}_j)},$$

which completes the proof.      □

Next, the key step is to find the expression for $\Pr(\mathscr{C}_k)$. To that end, we firstly define $\tau$ as the probability of nodes attempting to transmit in a randomly chosen time slot. And denote by $\mathscr{P}_j$ the event of losing a preamble or an ACK at time index $j$ due to collisions. Thus $\Pr(\bar{\mathscr{P}}_j) = 1 - (1 - \tau)^{M-1}$ is the probability that at least one of the remaining nodes attempts to transmit in the same time slot, where $M$ is the total number of nodes in once concurrent traffic load. As the size of a preamble and an ACK is much smaller, we assume that these probabilities are independent at each attempt.

Furthermore, let $\mathscr{D}_k$ as the event that the sink transmits $k$ preambles before the expiration of $T_p$. Denote by $\mathscr{F}_k$ as the event that an ACK message is transmitted successfully before timeout of the sink in case that $\mathscr{D}_k$ is true. Let $\Omega$ be the certain event. Now we are ready to determine $\Pr(\mathscr{C}_k)$ in Lemma 3.3.

**Lemma 3.3** *Following the definition of $\mathscr{C}_k$, it holds that*

$$\mathscr{C}_k = (\mathscr{D}_{k-1}\bar{\mathscr{F}}_{k-1} + \mathscr{D}_{k-1}\mathscr{F}_{k-1}\mathscr{P}_1)\mathscr{D}_k\mathscr{F}_k\bar{\mathscr{P}}_2, \tag{3.4}$$

*where*

$$\mathscr{D}_0 = \Omega, \quad \mathscr{D}_k = (kT_1 + (k - 1)\mathbb{1}_{(k-1)\geq 0}T_{out}) \leq T_p),$$

$$\bar{\mathscr{F}}_0 = (T_{ack} > T_{out}), \; \mathscr{F}_k = (T_{ack} \leq T_{out} |\mathscr{D}_k),$$

$$\bar{\mathscr{F}}_{k-1} = (T_{ack} > T_{out} |\mathscr{D}_{k-1}\mathbb{1}_{(k-1)\geq 0}).$$

*Proof* From the definition of $\mathscr{C}_k$, $\mathscr{C}_k$ consists of two events: (1) the event $\mathscr{C}_{1,k} = \mathscr{D}_{k-1}\bar{\mathscr{F}}_{k-1}\mathscr{D}_k\mathscr{F}_k\bar{\mathscr{P}}_2$ occurs when the $k - 1$th preamble was sent but the nodes were not able to send back an ACK before the timeout of the sink; and (2) the event $\mathscr{C}_{2,k} = \mathscr{D}_{k-1}\mathscr{F}_{k-1}\mathscr{P}_1\mathscr{D}_k\mathscr{F}_k\bar{\mathscr{P}}_2$ occurs when the $k - 1$th preamble was sent and an ACK was sent back before timeout but it was collided. As $\mathscr{C}_{1,k}\mathscr{C}_{2,k} = \phi$, we thus have

$$\Pr(\mathscr{C}_k) = \Pr(\mathscr{C}_{1,k}) + \Pr(\mathscr{C}_{2,k}). \tag{3.5}$$

Subsequently, we derive the probabilities of $\mathscr{C}_{1,k}$ and $\mathscr{C}_{2,k}$. By considering that the event of $\mathscr{F}_k$ and $\mathscr{P}_j$ is independent of the others, the probability of $\mathscr{C}_{1,k}$ is given as

$$\Pr(\mathscr{C}_{1,k}) = \Pr(\mathscr{D}_{k-1}\mathscr{D}_k) \Pr(\bar{\mathscr{F}}_{k-1}\mathscr{F}_k) \Pr(\bar{\mathscr{P}}_2),$$

for $\mathscr{D}_{k-1}\mathscr{D}_k = \mathscr{D}_k$. Since $\bar{\mathscr{F}}_{k-1}$ and $\mathscr{F}_k$ are independent, and $\Pr(\bar{\mathscr{F}}_{k-1}) = 1 - \Pr(\mathscr{F}_{k-1}) = 1 - \Pr(T_{ack} \leq T_{out})$, we have

$$\Pr(\mathscr{C}_{1,k}) = \Pr(\mathscr{D}_k) \Pr(\bar{\mathscr{F}}_{k-1}) \Pr(\mathscr{F}_k) \Pr(\bar{\mathscr{P}}_2)$$

$$= \Pr\left(kT_1 + (k - 1)T_{out} \leq T_p\right)(1 - \Pr(T_{ack} \leq T_{out})) \Pr(T_{ack} \leq T_{out})$$

$$\times \Pr(\bar{\mathscr{P}}_2). \tag{3.6}$$

Furthermore, since $\mathscr{D}_{k-1}\mathscr{D}_k = \mathscr{D}_k$ and $\mathscr{F}_{k-1}$ is independent of $\mathscr{F}_k$, it holds that

$$\mathscr{D}_{k-1}\mathscr{F}_{k-1}\mathscr{P}_1\mathscr{D}_k\mathscr{F}_k\bar{\mathscr{P}}_2 = \mathscr{F}_{k-1}\mathscr{P}_1\mathscr{D}_k\mathscr{F}_k\bar{\mathscr{P}}_2.$$

As a consequence, we can derive that

$$\begin{aligned}
\Pr(\mathscr{C}_{2,k}) &= \Pr(\mathscr{F}_{k-1})\Pr(\mathscr{D}_k)\Pr(\mathscr{F}_k)\Pr(\mathscr{P}_1)\Pr(\bar{\mathscr{P}}_2) \\
&= \Pr\left(kT_1 + (k-1)T_{out} \leq T_p\right)\Pr(T_{ack} \leq T_{out})^2\Pr(\mathscr{P}_1)\Pr(\bar{\mathscr{P}}_2).
\end{aligned}$$
(3.7)

Thus, substituting Eqs. (3.6)–(3.7) into Eq. (3.5) yields $\Pr(\mathscr{C}_k)$.      $\square$

As a result, the random delay in case 1 is $T_w = T_a + T_b$ as shown in Fig. 3.3.

*Case 2* The sink is awake when the node has a packet to transmit, as shown in the Fig. 3.4.

Inspired by the analysis in case 1, let $T_a'$ be the time interval between the wake-up instants of the sink and the node. From the definition of event $\mathscr{B}$, it holds that $T_a' = 0\mathbb{1}_{\mathscr{B}} + T_3\mathbb{1}_{\bar{\mathscr{B}}}$, where $T_3$ is the random time spent by the sink on waiting for the wakeup of the node given that the event $\mathscr{B}$ is false. Since $T_3$ has a uniform distribution in the range $[0, T_p]$, the probability mass function of $T_a'$ is

$$\Pr(T_a') = \begin{cases} \dfrac{T_{on}}{T_p(T_{on}+T_s)} & 0 < T_a' \leq T_p, \\[2ex] \dfrac{T_s}{T_{on}+T_s} & T_a' = 0. \end{cases}$$

Correspondingly, let $T_b'$ denote the random delay spent by the sink from its wake-up moment until a successful reception of one preamble given that the event $\bar{\mathscr{B}}$ is true. Referring to the derivation of $T_b$, $T_b'$ can be formulated as

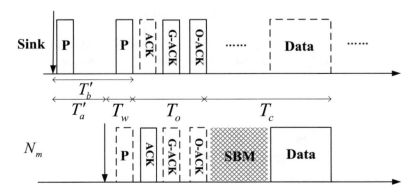

**Fig. 3.4** The sink is awake when the nodes wake up

$$T_b' = \sum_{k=1}^{N_p} \left( \sum_{j=1}^{k} T_{1,k,j} + (k-1)T_{out} \right) \mathbb{1}_{\mathscr{C}_k \mid \mathscr{C}}, \tag{3.8}$$

Note that the occurrence of $\mathscr{C}_k$ occurring in case 2 is different with that in case 1 since the sink does not know when the node wakes up. Although the expression of $T_b'$ is the same with $T_b$, the expression of $\Pr(\mathscr{C}_k)$ in case 2 differs from that in case 1, as shown in the following Lemma 3.4.

**Lemma 3.4** *In case 2, $\Pr(\mathscr{C}_k)$ is derived as*

$$\Pr(\mathscr{C}_k) = (\Pr(\mathscr{N}_k \mathscr{D}_k) - \Pr(\bar{\mathscr{E}}_k)) \Pr(\mathscr{F}_k) \Pr(\bar{\mathscr{P}}_2)$$

$$+ (\Pr(\mathscr{D}_k) - \Pr(\mathscr{N}_k \mathscr{D}_k)) \Pr(\bar{\mathscr{F}}_{k-1}) \Pr(\mathscr{F}_k) \Pr(\bar{\mathscr{P}}_2)$$

$$+ (\Pr(\mathscr{D}_k) - \Pr(\mathscr{N}_k \mathscr{D}_k)) \Pr(\bar{\mathscr{F}}_{k-1}) \Pr(\mathscr{F}_k) \Pr(\mathscr{P}_1) \Pr(\bar{\mathscr{P}}_2),$$

*where*

$$\Pr(\bar{\mathscr{E}}_k) = P_1 \left( \frac{T_a' - (k-1)T_{out}}{k} \right),$$

$$\Pr(\mathscr{D}_k) = P_1 \left( \frac{T_p - (k-1)T_{out}}{k} \right),$$

$$\Pr(\mathscr{N}_k) = P_1 \left( \frac{T_a' - (k-2)T_{out}}{k-1} \right),$$

$$\Pr(\mathscr{N}_k \mathscr{D}_k) = \Pr(\mathscr{D}_k) \left( 1 - \Pr(T_1 \le T_p - T_a' - T_{out}) \right)$$

$$+ \Pr(\mathscr{N}_k) \Pr(T_1 \le T_p - T_a' - T_{out}).$$

*Proof* Let $\mathscr{N}_k$ define the event occurring when the $k-1$th preamble is sent but the node is sleeping. And event $\mathscr{E}_k$ occurs when the $k$th preamble is sent and the node has woken up. Recall the definitions in case 1, we then have

$$\mathscr{C}_k = (\mathscr{N}_k + \mathscr{E}_{k-1} \mathscr{D}_{k-1} \bar{\mathscr{F}}_{k-1} + \mathscr{E}_{k-1} \mathscr{D}_{k-1} \bar{\mathscr{F}}_{k-1} \mathscr{P}_1) \mathscr{E}_k \mathscr{D}_k \mathscr{F}_k \bar{\mathscr{P}}_2,$$

where

$$\mathscr{N}_k = ((k-1)\mathbb{1}_{(k-1)\ge 0} T_1 + (k-2)\mathbb{1}_{(k-2)\ge 0} T_{out} \le T_a'),$$

$$\mathscr{E}_k = (kT_1 + (k-1)\mathbb{1}_{(k-1)\ge 0} T_{out} > T_a').$$

In case 2, a preamble fails in three situations, which follows that $\mathscr{C}_k = \mathscr{C}_{1,k} + \mathscr{C}_{2,k} + \mathscr{C}_{3,k}$, where $\mathscr{C}_{1,k} = \mathscr{N}_k \mathscr{E}_k \mathscr{D}_k \mathscr{F}_k \bar{\mathscr{P}}_2$ is the event that the node is sleeping when the sink sent the $k-1$th preamble; $\mathscr{C}_{2,k} = \mathscr{E}_{k-1} \mathscr{D}_{k-1} \bar{\mathscr{F}}_{k-1} \mathscr{E}_k \mathscr{D}_k \mathscr{F}_k \bar{\mathscr{P}}_2$ is the event occurring when the $k-1$th preamble was sent but the corresponding ACK is not sent back before the timeout; and $\mathscr{C}_{3,k} = \mathscr{E}_{k-1}\mathscr{D}_{k-1}\mathscr{F}_{k-1}\mathscr{P}_1\mathscr{E}_k\mathscr{D}_k\mathscr{F}_k\bar{\mathscr{P}}_2$ is the event that the $k-1$th ACK sent back before timeout was collided. For $\mathscr{C}_{1,k}$, $\mathscr{C}_{2,k}$ and $\mathscr{C}_{3,k}$ are mutually exclusive, we have

$$\Pr(\mathscr{C}_k) = \Pr(\mathscr{C}_{1,k}) + \Pr(\mathscr{C}_{2,k}) + \Pr(\mathscr{C}_{3,k}). \tag{3.9}$$

Hence, the key is to derive $\Pr(\mathscr{C}_{1,k})$, $\Pr(\mathscr{C}_{2,k})$, and $\Pr(\mathscr{C}_{3,k})$.

For the mutual independence of the event $\mathscr{F}_k$ and $\mathscr{P}_j$, the probability of $\mathscr{C}_{1,k}$ is given by

$$\Pr(\mathscr{C}_{1,k}) = \Pr(\mathscr{N}_k\mathscr{E}_k\mathscr{D}_k)\Pr(\mathscr{F}_k)\bar{\mathscr{P}}_2.$$

Following the total probability theorem, we have

$$\Pr(\mathscr{N}_k\mathscr{D}_k) = \Pr(\mathscr{N}_k\mathscr{E}_k\mathscr{D}_k) + \Pr(\mathscr{N}_k\bar{\mathscr{E}}_k\mathscr{D}_k),$$

and it holds that $\mathscr{N}_k\bar{\mathscr{E}}_k\mathscr{D}_k = \bar{\mathscr{E}}_k\mathscr{D}_k = \bar{\mathscr{E}}_k$, such that

$$\Pr(\mathscr{N}_k\mathscr{E}_k\mathscr{D}_k) = \Pr(\mathscr{N}_k\mathscr{D}_k) - \Pr(\bar{\mathscr{E}}_k). \tag{3.10}$$

Rewriting $\mathscr{N}_k$ as $\mathscr{N}_k = kT_1 + (k-1)T_{out} \leq T'_a + T_1 + T_{out}$, we have

$$\mathscr{N}_k\mathscr{D}_k = \begin{cases} \mathscr{D}_k & \text{if } T_p \leq T'_a + T_1 + T_{out} \\ \mathscr{N}_k & \text{otherwise} \end{cases}$$

whereby

$$\Pr(\mathscr{N}_k\mathscr{D}_k) = \Pr(\mathscr{D}_k)(1 - \Pr(T_1 \leq T_p - T'_a - T_{out})) + \Pr(\mathscr{N}_k)\Pr(T_1 \leq T_p - T'_a - T_{out}).$$

Combining this with Eq. (3.10) yields

$$\Pr(\mathscr{C}_{1,k}) = (\Pr(\mathscr{N}_k\mathscr{D}_k) - \Pr(\bar{\mathscr{E}}_k))\Pr(\mathscr{F}_k)\Pr(\bar{\mathscr{P}}_2). \tag{3.11}$$

We next compute $\Pr(\mathscr{C}_{2,k})$, because $\mathscr{E}_{k-1}\mathscr{E}_k = \mathscr{E}_{k-1} = \bar{\mathscr{N}}_k$ and $\mathscr{D}_{k-1}\mathscr{D}_k = \mathscr{D}_k$, we have

$$\mathscr{E}_{k-1}\mathscr{D}_{k-1}\bar{\mathscr{F}}_{k-1}\mathscr{E}_k\mathscr{D}_k\mathscr{F}_k\bar{\mathscr{P}}_2 = \mathscr{E}_{k-1}\mathscr{D}_k\bar{\mathscr{F}}_{k-1}\mathscr{F}_k\bar{\mathscr{P}}_2.$$

Moreover, $\bar{\mathscr{F}}_{k-1}$ and $\mathscr{F}_k$ are independent, so it holds that

$$\begin{aligned} \Pr(\mathscr{C}_{2,k}) &= \Pr(\bar{\mathscr{N}}_k\mathscr{D}_k)\Pr(\bar{\mathscr{F}}_{k-1})\Pr(\mathscr{F}_k)\Pr(\bar{\mathscr{P}}_2) \\ &= (\Pr(\mathscr{D}_k) - \Pr(\mathscr{N}_k\mathscr{D}_k))\Pr(\bar{\mathscr{F}}_{k-1})\Pr(\mathscr{F}_k)\Pr(\bar{\mathscr{P}}_2). \end{aligned} \tag{3.12}$$

Similarly, we have

$$\mathscr{E}_{k-1}\mathscr{D}_{k-1}\mathscr{F}_{k-1}\mathscr{P}_1\mathscr{E}_k\mathscr{D}_k\mathscr{F}_k\bar{\mathscr{P}}_2 = \mathscr{E}_{k-1}\mathscr{D}_k\mathscr{F}_{k-1}\mathscr{P}_1\mathscr{F}_k\bar{\mathscr{P}}_2.$$

Correspondingly, we can derive that

$$\begin{aligned}
\Pr(\mathscr{C}_{3,k}) &= \Pr(\bar{\mathscr{N}_k}\mathscr{D}_k)\Pr(\mathscr{F}_{k-1})\Pr(\mathscr{P}_1)\Pr(\mathscr{F}_k)\Pr(\bar{\mathscr{P}}_2)\\
&=(\Pr(\mathscr{D}_k)-\Pr(\mathscr{N}_k\mathscr{D}_k))\Pr(\mathscr{F}_{k-1})\Pr(\mathscr{F}_k)\Pr(\mathscr{P}_1)\Pr(\bar{\mathscr{P}}_2).
\end{aligned} \tag{3.13}$$

Therefore, incorporating Eqs. (3.11)–(3.13) leads to $\Pr(\mathscr{C}_k)$ in case 2.  □

Consequently, the delay in case 2 is $T_w = T_b' - T_a'$ as shown in Fig. 3.4. In summary, since $T_w$ is given by the weighted sum of variables approximated as Gaussian distributed in Sect. 3.6.1, it follows that $T_w$ can also be approximated by a Gaussian random variable.

### 3.6.3 Modeling of $T_o$ and $T_c$

In this section we analyze $T_o$ and $T_c$, which are defined as the random delay spent by the node from the reception of a preamble until the reception of the O-ACK and from the O-ACK reception until the transmission of a packet, respectively. We assume that concurrent traffic load comes from $M$ nodes, and $N_m$ represents the node that $m$thly sends data packet.

In order to receive all probable ACKs from concurrent active nodes, the sink needs to send G-ACK to the nodes multiple times. Let $N_a$ and $N_o$ be the maximum numbers of G-ACK and O-ACK that can be sent by the sink, respectively. Denote by $\mathscr{R}_n$ as the event that the sink has to send $n$ G-ACKs until no ACK from nodes is received. And denote by $\mathscr{Q}_l$ as the event that the $l$th O-ACK is received successfully by the nodes. According to the aforementioned analysis on $T_b$ and $T_b'$, we can formulate the random delay of $T_o$ as

$$\begin{aligned}
T_o = \sum_{k=1}^{N_p}\Bigg(\sum_{n=1}^{N_a}\Bigg(\sum_{i=1}^{n}(T_{out}+T_{gack,n,i})+T_{out}\\
+\sum_{l=1}^{N_o}\sum_{j=1}^{l}(T_{oack,l,j}+T_{SIFS})\mathbb{1}_{\mathscr{Q}_l|\mathscr{Q}}\Bigg)\mathbb{1}_{\mathscr{R}_n|\mathscr{R}}\Bigg)\mathbb{1}_{\mathscr{C}_k|\mathscr{C}},
\end{aligned} \tag{3.14}$$

where $T_{gack,n,i}$ is the random delay to transmit the $i$th G-ACK when the O-ACK is sent after the $n$th G-ACK transmission. And $\mathscr{R}$ is the event that the sink receives all ACKs within $N_a$ transmissions of G-ACK. Correspondingly, $T_{oack,l,j}$ is the delay to transmit the $j$th O-ACK when the $l$th O-ACK is received successfully by the nodes. And $\mathscr{Q}$ is the event that the O-ACK is received successfully within $N_o$ transmissions. $T_{SIFS}$ is the short interframe space interval among the separated data packet transmission. Note that the probabilities of $\mathscr{R}_n$ and $\mathscr{Q}_l$ can be calculated by the same method as that of $\mathscr{C}_k$. In the sake of the limited space, the probabilistic characteristics of $T_o$ are omitted, which can refer to Lemma 3.2.

Then, the delay to accomplish the data transmission for the node $N_m$ can be approximated as

$$T_{c_m} = \sum_{k=1}^{N_p} \sum_{n=1}^{N_a} \sum_{l=1}^{N_o} m \cdot (T_{SIFS} + T_{data}) \mathbb{1}_{\mathscr{Q}_l | \mathscr{Q}} \mathbb{1}_{\mathscr{R}_n | \mathscr{R}} \mathbb{1}_{\mathscr{L}_k | \mathscr{C}},$$

where $T_{data}$ is the delay to transmit one packet, i.e., $T_{data} = L_p/R_s + T_{hr}$, where $L_p$ is the payload of one packet in bits and $R_s$ is data rate in bits/s as in IEEE 802.15.6 [25], and $T_{hr}$ is the time taken by the hardware platform to process the packet and propagate it. In fact, $T_{c_m}$ consists of $(m-1)(T_{SIFS} + T_{data})$ when the node stays in SBM and one $(T_{SIFS} + T_{data})$ when the node sends a data packet.

Therefore, the delay for the successful communication between the sink and a node is given by $T_d = T_w + T_o + T_c$, which can be approximated by a Gaussian distribution with mean $\mu_{T_d} = \mu_{T_w} + \mu_{T_o} + \mu_{T_c}$ and variance $\sigma_{T_d}^2 = \sigma_{T_w}^2 + \sigma_{T_o}^2 + \sigma_{T_c}^2$.

### 3.6.4  Accuracy Evaluation

In this section, we evaluate the accuracy of the theoretical analysis. In the simulation, we assume that all nodes have the same user priority $U_p$. The detail numerical and simulation parameters are listed in Table 3.3.

Figures 3.5 and 3.6 illustrate the analytic and emulational expectation and variance of the transmission delay $T_d$ for a network with 10 nodes and traffic arrival rate $\lambda = 0.02$ as a function of the sleep time $T_s$ and active time $T_{on}$, respectively. As shown in figures, the theoretical results match well with the simulation results, verifying the accuracy of the theoretical analysis. Moreover, a good linear relationship between delay and the sleep time can be inferred from Fig. 3.5, especially in the case that $T_{on} \leq T_s$, since the packet transmission time and the active time are very short compared to the sleep time. And this trend is

**Table 3.3** Simulation settings

| Parameter | Value | Parameter | Value | Parameter | Value |
|---|---|---|---|---|---|
| $R_s$ | 242.9 kbps | $T_{hr}$ | 1 μs | $CW_{min}$ | 2 |
| $S_p$ | 88 bits/$R_s$ | $T_{SIFS}$ | 75 μs | $CW_{max}$ | 8 |
| $L_p$ | 255 bytes | $L_{ack}$ | 11 bytes | $N_b$ | 5 |
| $P_{rx}$ | 96.6 mW | $S_b$ | 125 μs | $N_p$ | 10 |
| $P_{tx}$ | 86.2 mW | $P_s$ | 1.6 mW | $N_a, N_o$ | 10,10 |

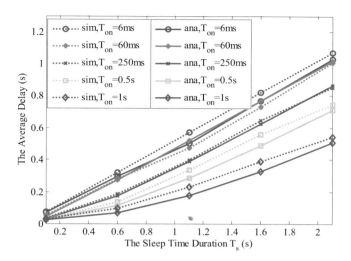

**Fig. 3.5** The expectation of $T_d$

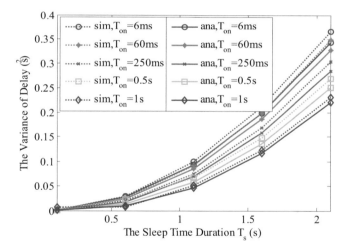

**Fig. 3.6** The variance of $T_d$

similar to that reported in [28]. Moreover, the average delay decreases as the active duration increases, but it is at the cost of more energy consumption of the sink which will be analyzed in the following performance evaluation Sect. 3.8.

## 3.7  Energy Consumption Analysis

In this section, we formulate the upper bound of the total normalized energy consumption of the network under C-MAC protocol described in Sect. 3.5.

### 3.7.1  Modeling of Energy Consumption

Since the energy consumed per unit time is rather low in the sleep state, we thus focus on the energy consumption spent in the active state. As a result, the total normalized energy consumption of the network per unit time is given by

$$E_{total} = \sum_{m=1}^{M} \frac{E_{N_m}}{T_{d_m}} + \frac{E_{sink}}{T_{on}} \tag{3.15}$$

where $E_{N_m}$ and $T_{d_m}$ are the energy consumption and random delay spent by the node $N_m$ to successfully transmit a packet, respectively, and $E_{sink}$ is the energy consumption spent by the sink in its whole active state. The energy consumption per node is normalized by its active duration to obtain the average energy consumption per unit time. The energy components $E_{N_m}$ and $E_{sink}$ are formulated in the following Lemma 3.5.

**Lemma 3.5** *According to the delay analysis in Sect. 3.6, the total energy consumption for the sink and the node $N_m$ are upper bounded as*

$$E_{sink} \leq \sum_{i=1}^{N_p} \left( \sum_{n=1}^{i} E_{tx,T_1}^n + (i-1)E_{T_{out}} + E_{T_o} + M E_{rx,T_{data}} \right) \mathbb{1}_{\mathscr{C}_i} \tag{3.16}$$

$$+ \left( \sum_{n=1}^{N_p} E_{tx,T_1}^n + N_p E_{T_{out}} \right) \mathbb{1}_{\bar{\mathscr{C}}}$$

$$E_{N_m} \leq E_{rx,p} + E_{T_o} + E_{SBM} + E_{tx,T_{data}} \tag{3.17}$$

*where $\bar{\mathscr{C}} = \bigcap_{i=1}^{N_p} \bar{\mathscr{C}_i}$ and*

$$E_{tx,T_1}^n = \sum_{k=1}^{N_b} \left( \sum_{j=1}^{k} P_{rx} \cdot t_{p,k,j} + P_{tx} \cdot S_p \right) \mathbb{1}_{\mathscr{A}_k}, \tag{3.18}$$

$$E_{T_{out}} = P_{rx} \cdot T_{out}, \tag{3.19}$$

$$E_{T_o} \leq max(P_{tx}, P_{rx})T_o, \tag{3.20}$$

$$E_{rx,T_{data}} = P_{rx}(T_{SIFS} + T_{data}), \tag{3.21}$$

$$E_{tx,T_{data}} = P_{tx}(T_{SIFS} + T_{data}), \tag{3.22}$$

$$E_{rx,p} \leq P_{rx}T_w + P_{rx}S_p, \tag{3.23}$$

$$E_{SBM} = (m - 1)P_s(T_{data} + T_{SIFS}), \tag{3.24}$$

where $P_s$ is the power consumed in SBM, $P_{tx}$ and $P_{rx}$ are the energy dissipated to transmit and receive packet, respectively. And $S_p$ is the preamble packet duration.

*Proof* The upper bound of $E_{sink}$ is the sum of two main components: one corresponding to the case that data packet transmissions are successful, and the other corresponding to the case that no data packet transmission is successful.

The $i$th term in the first component corresponds to the case where the $i$th preamble is successfully transmitted and the corresponding ACKs are received from nodes, i.e., $\mathbb{1}_{\mathscr{C}_i} = 1$. In this case, the energy consumption consists of four parts:

- For the first part, the energy spent for the preamble transmission is given by the sum from the 1st preamble to the $i$th preamble, i.e., $\sum_{n=1}^{i} E_{tx,T_1}^n$. Recall the analysis of $T_1$ in Sect. 3.6.1, the energy consumption spent by the sink on backoff and the transmission of the $n$th preamble can be expressed as Eq. (3.18), where each term of the sum with respect to $k$ corresponds to the case that the channel is busy in the first $k - 1$ times and idle at the $k$th trial.
- For the second part, we define the energy spent in waiting for the ACKs following each preamble transmission as $E_{T_{out}}$, its expression is given in Eq. (3.19). Thus, the energy wastage during the timeout periods for the first $i - 1$ preambles can be calculated as $(i - 1)E_{T_{out}}$.
- For the third part, the energy used to receive the corresponding ACKs and broadcast the G-ACKs and O-ACKs is great difficult to give a closed-form expression, as it depends on the actual transmission numbers of G-ACKs and O-ACKs. We thus provide an upper bound of $E_{T_o}$ given in Eq. (3.20) following the analysis of $T_o$ in Sect. 3.6.3 to simply the analysis.
- For the fourth part, the energy dissipated to receive the subsequent $M$ packets is $ME_{rx,T_{data}}$, where $E_{rx,T_{data}}$ is shown in Eq. (3.21).

The second component corresponds to the case where all the preambles are not received successfully, thus, the energy consumption in this case equals to the energy spent transmitting $N_p$ preambles and waiting for $N_p$ timeouts.

Furthermore, for the node $N_m$, the upper boundary of the energy consumption is derived as in Eq. (3.17), which is also composed of four parts. Note that the part of $E_{T_o}$ here is the same with that of the sink. Denote by $E_{rx,p}$ the energy used for successfully receiving a preamble from the sink, we bound $E_{rx,p}$ upwards as in Eq. (3.23) following the modeling of $T_w$ in Sect. 3.6.2. Moreover, $E_{SBM}$ is the energy dissipation during the SBM state which can be expressed as Eq. (3.24).

Besides, $E_{tx, T_{data}}$, defining the energy spent by the node on transmitting a packet, is formulated in Eq. (3.22).                                                                                    □

*Remark* Because the node has to listen to the channel status during the backoff and timeout duration, the power consumption is assumed to equal to $P_{rx}$.

Since the events involved in the calculation of $E_{sink}$ and $E_{N_m}$ are highly cross correlated, it is very difficult to model the accurate characteristics of $E_{total}$. But we can compute the upper bound of $E_{total}$ by using Eq. (3.15) and Lemma 3.5.

### 3.7.2   Accuracy Evaluation

In this section, we validate the correctness of theoretical normalized energy consumption by comparing the analytical results with simulation results in different duty cycles.

Figure 3.7 shows the analytical and simulation results of the total normalized energy consumption in dB as a function of $T_s$ and $T_{on}$ for a network with 10 nodes and traffic arrival rate $\lambda = 0.02$. This figure shows a good matching of the analysis results with simulations, which further demonstrates the correctness of the mathematical analysis.

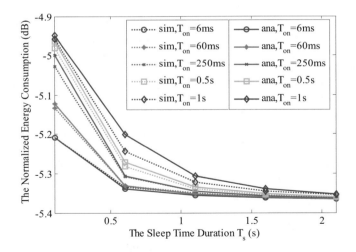

**Fig. 3.7**  The analytical and simulation results of $E_{total}$

## 3.8 Performance Evaluation

In the previous sections, we have formulated the delay and energy consumption and validated the analysis accuracy by numerical and simulation results. In this section, we further evaluate the performance of C-MAC protocol by comparing with two recent receiver-initiated protocols: RI-MAC [18] and A-MAC [19].

### 3.8.1 Simulation Settings

The parameters in the simulation are set in accordance with the data sheet of CC2420 radio chip [29] which is used in popular motes, and the specifications in the IEEE 802.15.6 standard [25] at 2.4 GHZ. We summarize the parameters in Table 3.3. Moreover, each simulation result is computed by the average of 100 independent experiments.

### 3.8.2 Simulation Results and Analysis

In this section, we present the simulation results and evaluate the performance of C-MAC.

**(1) Delay** Here, we show the average delay of each node in Figs. 3.8 and 3.9.

In order to better assess the impact of the concurrent traffic on the delay, we plot the average delay of each node with the number of nodes $M = 5, 10$ and the traffic arrival rate $\lambda = 0.02, 0.2$, respectively, in Fig. 3.8. As shown in these figures, the average delay of C-MAC is much smaller than that of RI-MAC and A-MAC in every case, especially for the later nodes. Moreover, a quantitative comparison can be made from Fig. 3.8a and b that C-MAC can reduce 18.12% and 22.54% of the average delay of RI-MAC, and 14.94% and 19.11% of that of A-MAC as packet arrival rate $\lambda = 0.02$ and $\lambda = 0.2$, respectively. Similarly, as shown in Fig. 3.8c and d, C-MAC outperforms RI-MAC over $-26.76\%$ and $-31.11\%$, and A-MAC over $-22.11\%$ and $-27.43\%$ in average delay.

The reason for the high delay of RI-MAC and A-MAC is that they do not take preventive measures to avoid collisions. Due to the numerous collisions under concurrent traffic load, data packets in RI-MAC and A-MAC are retransmitted frequently, resulting in the large delay. In contrast, C-MAC employs CSMA/CA mechanism, which can tremendously reduce the collision probability in advance. Moreover, sequencing data packet transmission can completely eradicate the collision in the second phase. Thereby, C-MAC can greatly reduce the additional delay caused by the collisions.

In addition, we can find that C-MAC can achieve high adaptivity for dynamic concurrent traffic load in WBSNs. For example, when the traffic arrival rate increases from 0.02 to 0.2, the delay of RI-MAC and A-MAC increases by 7.17%

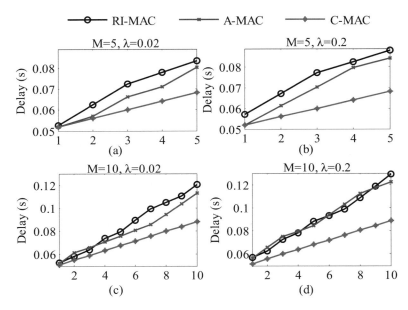

**Fig. 3.8** The average delay with different traffic loads. (**a–d**) $N_\mathrm{m}$

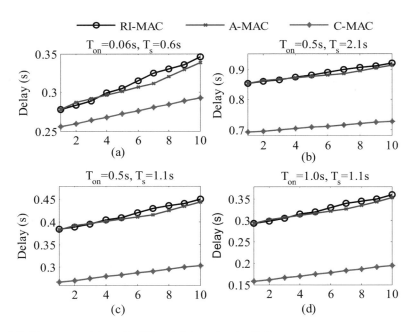

**Fig. 3.9** The average delay with different duty cycles. (**a–d**) $N_\mathrm{m}$

and 8.17% while that of C-MAC only increases by 0.79%. Note that the same conclusion can also be drawn for the different number of nodes.

In order to better evaluate the influence of the duty cycle on the delay, Fig. 3.9 shows the simulation results of C-MAC, A-MAC, and RI-MAC with respective to different percentages of $T_{on}$, i.e., about 10%, 20%, 30%, and 50% for a WBSN with 10 nodes and traffic arrival rate $\lambda = 0.02$.

As depicted in Fig. 3.9, C-MAC can achieve much smaller delay than RI-MAC and A-MAC in every case. Specially, the enhancement of C-MAC can reach to at least about 15.31%, 20.84%, 32.64%, and 46.13% over RI-MAC and A-MAC, respectively, by comparing Fig. 3.9a–d.

In other words, with the increase of the proportion of $T_{on}$, the improvement of C-MAC becomes more and more significant. Furthermore, even under light traffic load, the C-MAC can also outperform RI-MAC and A-MAC, which further verifies the adaptivity of C-MAC.

Consequently, C-MAC shows better delay performance than RI-MAC and A-MAC.

**(2) Energy Consumption** We here show the energy consumption of C-MAC.

Since A-MAC is more energy-efficient than RI-MAC [19], for the sake of clarity, we just compare C-MAC with A-MAC temporally. Figure 3.10 presents the total normalized energy consumption of the whole network with $M = 5$ and $\lambda = 0.02$. We can see that C-MAC is more energy-efficient than A-MAC, especially, as the sleep duration $T_s$ is small. The lower energy consumption of C-MAC can be attributed to its great capacity of reducing collisions, idle listening, and overhearing.

Moreover, in order to better understand the energy consumption of C-MAC, we further plot the normalized energy consumption for each node in Fig. 3.11.

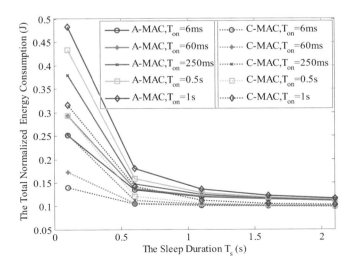

**Fig. 3.10** The whole network NEC

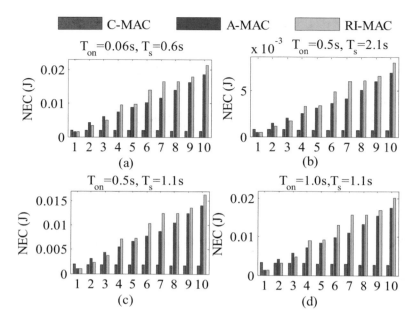

**Fig. 3.11** The NEC of each node. (**a–d**) $N_m$

Note that for the limited space in subgraphs, the normalized energy consumption is abbreviated as NEC.

We can obtain two main observations from Fig. 3.11. First, the NEC of each node in C-MAC is much smaller than that in RI-MAC and A-MAC. Second, the energy budget to transmit a packet in C-MAC is almost the same for each node, while the later transmission for a node, the more energy budget in RI-MAC and A-MAC. The main reasons are twofold. First, in RI-MAC and A-MAC, the nodes must keep active until its packet is transmitted successfully. Thus, the later nodes need persistently to listen to the channel and may overhear other nodes' packets, wasting much energy. Second, in C-MAC, they can switch to SBM until their individual turn, avoiding idle listening and overhearing.

Furthermore, a quantitative comparison can be made from Fig. 3.11 that C-MAC mostly outperforms RI-MAC and A-MAC over 90.42%, 89.46%, 87.88%, and 84.85% in every duty cycle, respectively. Therefore, we can conclude that C-MAC not only reduces the energy consumption of the network but also lowers and balances the energy budget for each node.

However, the improvement in energy consumption of each node is at the cost of the more energy consumption of the sink, as shown in Fig. 3.12. The main reason is that C-MAC is a receiver-initiated protocol that the preambles must be sent periodically by the sink as it wakes up. Besides, the sink must persistently listen to the channel after transmitting a preamble to detect if there are incoming packets.

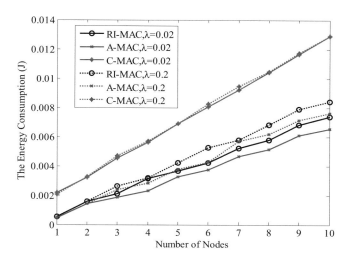

**Fig. 3.12** The normalized energy consumption of the sink

In addition, in order to receive all probable ACKs from nodes, the sink has to send G-ACKs multiple times.

Furthermore, as in Fig. 3.12, the energy consumption of the sink is almost not influenced by traffic arrival rate, which further demonstrates the strong adaptiveness of C-MAC to the concurrent traffic load.

From all these results, we can conclude that C-MAC is able to effectively and efficiently reduce delay and conserve energy, especially under concurrent traffic.

## 3.9  Conclusion

This chapter addressed the delay and energy consumption under concurrent traffic in the medical applications of WBSNs. To that end, we designed and analyzed a two-phase receiver-initiated asynchronous duty-cycling protocol, called C-MAC.

In the first phase, C-MAC employs the IEEE 802.15.6 CSMA/CA mechanism to avoid collisions and sequenced the data packet transmission of different nodes to resolve collisions in the second phase. Moreover, C-MAC enables nodes to switch to SBM in the second phase, which dramatically reduces the idle listening and overhearing. Subsequently, we derive the mathematical expressions of delay and energy consumption and further verified their correctness by the numerical analysis and simulation. Furthermore, extensive simulations results demonstrate that the performance of C-MAC outperforms RI-MAC and A-MAC, especially for concurrent traffic.

# References

1. S. González-Valenzuela, M. Chen, V.C. Leung, Mobility support for health monitoring at home using wearable sensors. IEEE Trans. Inf. Technol. Biomed. **15**(4), 539–549 (2011)
2. M. Patel, J. Wang, Applications, challenges, and prospective in emerging body area networking technologies. IEEE Wirel. Commun. Mag. **17**(1), 80–88 (2010)
3. S. Movassaghi, M. Abolhasan, J. Lipman, D. Smith, A. Jamalipour, Wireless body area networks: a survey. IEEE Commun. Surv. Tutorials **16**(3), 1658–1686 (2014)
4. N. Javaid, S. Hayat, M. Shakir, M. Khan, S.H. Bouk, Z. Khan, Energy efficient MAC protocols in wireless body area sensor networks-a survey (2013). Preprint. arXiv:1303.2072
5. S. Ullah, B. Shen, S. Riazul Islam, P. Khan, S. Saleem, K. Sup Kwak, A study of mac protocols for WBANs. Sensors **10**(1), 128–145 (2009)
6. A. Rai, S. Deswal, P. Singh, Mac protocols in wireless sensor network: a survey. Int. J. New Innov. Eng. Technol. **5**(1), 95–101 (2016)
7. K. Han, J. Luo, Y. Liu, A.V. Vasilakos, Algorithm design for data communications in duty-cycled wireless sensor networks: a survey. IEEE Commun. Mag. **51**(7), 107–113 (2013)
8. T. Van Dam, K. Langendoen, An adaptive energy-efficient MAC protocol for wireless sensor networks, in *Proceedings of the 1st International Conference on Embedded Networked Sensor Systems* (ACM, New York, 2003), pp. 171–180
9. S. Du, A.K. Saha, D.B. Johnson, RMAC: a routing-enhanced duty-cycle MAC protocol for wireless sensor networks, in *IEEE INFOCOM 2007-26th IEEE International Conference on Computer Communications* (IEEE, Piscataway, 2007), pp. 1478–1486
10. C.J. Merlin, W.B. Heinzelman, Schedule adaptation of low-power-listening protocols for wireless sensor networks. IEEE Trans. Mob. Comput. **9**(5), 672–685 (2010)
11. M.O. Rahman, C.S. Hong, S. Lee, Y.-C. Bang, ATLAS: A traffic load aware sensor MAC design for collaborative body area sensor networks. Sensors **11**(12), 11560–11580 (2011)
12. C. Beck, J. Nagel, P. Hevesi, G. Bretthauer, RTS-MAC: a relative time synchronization MAC protocol for low duty cycle body sensor networks. Int. J. Wireless Inf. Networks **19**(3), 163–172 (2012)
13. P. Sthapit, J.-Y. Pyun, Medium reservation based sensor MAC protocol for low latency and high energy efficiency. Telecommun. Syst. **52**(4), 2387–2395 (2013)
14. J. Polastre, J. Hill, D. Culler, Versatile low power media access for wireless sensor networks, in *Proceedings of the 2nd International Conference on Embedded Networked Sensor Systems* (ACM, New York, 2004), pp. 95–107
15. M. Buettner, G.V. Yee, E. Anderson, R. Han, X-MAC: a short preamble MAC protocol for duty-cycled wireless sensor networks, in *Proceedings of the 4th International Conference on Embedded Networked Sensor Systems* (ACM, New York, 2006), pp. 307–320
16. A. El-Hoiydi, J.-D. Decotignie, WiseMAC: An ultra low power MAC protocol for multi-hop wireless sensor networks, in *International Symposium on Algorithms and Experiments for Sensor Systems, Wireless Networks and Distributed Robotics* (Springer, Berlin, 2004), pp. 18–31
17. X. Fafoutis, A. Di Mauro, M.D. Vithanage, N. Dragoni, Receiver-initiated medium access control protocols for wireless sensor networks. Comput. Netw. **76**, 55–74 (2015)
18. Y. Sun, O. Gurewitz, D.B. Johnson, RI-MAC: a receiver-initiated asynchronous duty cycle MAC protocol for dynamic traffic loads in wireless sensor networks, in *Proceedings of the 6th ACM Conference on Embedded Network Sensor Systems* (ACM, New York, 2008), pp. 1–14
19. P. Dutta, S. Dawson-Haggerty, Y. Chen, C.-J.M. Liang, A. Terzis, Design and evaluation of a versatile and efficient receiver-initiated link layer for low-power wireless, in *Proceedings of the 8th ACM Conference on Embedded Networked Sensor Systems* (ACM, New York, 2010), pp. 1–14
20. L. Tang, Y. Sun, O. Gurewitz, D.B. Johnson, PW-MAC: an energy-efficient predictive-wakeup MAC protocol for wireless sensor networks, in *2011 Proceedings IEEE of INFOCOM* (IEEE, Piscataway, 2011), pp. 1305–1313

21. M.M. Alam, O. Berder, D. Menard, O. Sentieys, TAD-MAC: traffic-aware dynamic MAC protocol for wireless body area sensor networks. IEEE J. Emerging Sel. Top. Circuits Syst. **2**(1), 109–119 (2012)

22. P. Huang, C. Wang, L. Xiao, RC-MAC: a receiver-centric MAC protocol for event-driven wireless sensor networks. IEEE Trans. Comput. **64**(4), 1149–1161 (2015)

23. K. Tuck, *Low Power Modes and Auto-Wake/Sleep Using the MMA8450q* (2010), http://cache.freescale.com/files/sensors/doc/app_note/AN3921.pdf

24. Atmel Corporation, *AVR1010: Minimizing the Power Consumption of Atmel AVR XMEGA Devices* (2010), http://www.atmel.com/Images/doc8267.pdf.

25. I.S. Association et al., IEEE standard for local and metropolitan area networks-part 15.6: wireless body area networks. IEEE Stand. Inf. Technol. **802**(6), 1–271 (2012)

26. R.C. Carrano, D. Passos, L.C. Magalhaes, C.V. Albuquerque, Survey and taxonomy of duty cycling mechanisms in wireless sensor networks. IEEE Commun. Surv. Tutorials **16**(1), 181–194 (2014)

27. A. Maskooki, C.B. Soh, E. Gunawan, K.S. Low, Adaptive routing for dynamic on-body wireless sensor networks. IEEE J. Biomed. Health Inform. **19**(2), 549–558 (2015)

28. H. Lee, J. Hong, S. Yang, I. Jang, H. Yoon, A pseudo-random asynchronous duty cycle MAC protocol in wireless sensor networks. IEEE Commun. Lett. **14**(2), 136–138 (2010)

29. CC2420 Data Sheet, 2.4 GHz IEEE 802.15.4/ZigBee-ready RF transceiver (2014). http://www.ti.com/lit/ds/symlink/cc2420.pdf.

# Chapter 4
# Multi-Channel Broadcast Algorithms in Duty-Cycling WBSNs

**Chapter Roadmap** The rest of this chapter is organized as follows: Section 4.1 explains the motivation of studying multi-channel broadcast algorithm and summarizes the contributions. Section 4.2 gives a brief overview of related work in broadcast algorithms. Sections 4.3 and 4.4 formulate the multi-channel broadcast problem and establish the theoretical delay bound, respectively. In Sections 4.5 and 4.6, we show the design of MCB from the single-channel and multi-channel cases, respectively. And an improved MCB algorithm is further proposed in Sect. 4.7. The performance of our proposed algorithms is evaluated in Sect. 4.8. Finally, we conclude the chapter in Sect. 4.9.

## 4.1 Introduction

### 4.1.1 Context and Motivation

In WBSNs, broadcast that the sink disseminates the control message to all sensor nodes is an essential or fundamental operation for network configuration [1, 2], secure key management [3], and data collection [4–6]. Therefore, it is of practical importance to design reliable and efficient broadcast algorithm for WBSNs, which, however, is challenged by the characteristic of practical WBSNs.

Firstly, widely applied duty cycle operation mode in WBSNs differs the studied broadcast problem from the traditional one. Specifically, the sink and each sensor node in WBSNs work in duty cycle mode for energy conservation by alternating between the shorter active and the longer sleep states [7]. In a duty-cycling WBSN, the broadcast message can be delivered to a sensor node if and only if the sink and the sensor node wake up at the same time slot. But due to the asymmetry between the sink and sensor nodes depending on their independent energy constraint and individual applications, they may have asymmetrical desired duty cycles and

© Springer Nature Switzerland AG 2020
R. Zhang and J. Yu, *Energy-Efficient Algorithms and Protocols for Wireless Body Sensor Networks*, https://doi.org/10.1007/978-3-030-28580-7_4

may fail to activate in the same time slots, it is thus a challenging problem that how to schedule the wake-up slots while guaranteeing the required duty cycles and successful broadcast delivery without any prior coordination.

Moreover, the lack of clock synchronization makes the broadcast problem more difficult. Since it is extremely difficult to maintain tight synchronization among local clocks of the sink and the sensor nodes in a distributed system, their clocks may drift away from each other, which may lead to the broadcast failure even though they wake up in the same time slot number in the sense of their individual local clocks. Therefore, broadcast algorithm should operate efficiently even in WBSNs with asynchronous local clocks.

Furthermore, multi-channel communication pattern provides an additional dimension to the broadcast problem. To alleviate bandwidth limitations and improving throughput and reliability in wireless communications, the sink and sensor nodes are allowed to operate on multiple frequency channels as specified in IEEE 802.15.6 standard [8]. One fundamental question arises in such setting: how can the sink and sensor nodes hop to the same channel in the same time slot without prior knowledge of each other and without external assistance, which is the key point in the design of an effective broadcast algorithm. On the other hand, from the perspective of the notorious instability of wireless channels in both time and space domains, the sink and sensor nodes may experience different channel perceptions due to their locations, interference, and noises. Consequently, an effective broadcast algorithm needs also to guarantee the broadcast delivery between the sink and any sensor node on every common channel they can access, in order to achieve maximum robustness which is of great importance in the medical monitoring application of WBSNs.

Formally, the multi-channel broadcast problem can be formulated as:

**Problem 4.1 (Multi-Channel Broadcast Problem)** Consider a WBSN of one sink and multiple sensor nodes with asymmetric duty cycles, operating on different channels, without clock synchronization, how can the sink successfully broadcasts control information to all sensor nodes over every common channel within a bounded delay?

Particularly, the following requirements must be satisfied:

- Maximum broadcast diversity/reliability with bounded (and minimum) worst-case broadcast delay;
- Support for heterogeneous and arbitrary duty cycles with fine-grained control.

We emphasize that the combination of the above system settings and design requirements makes the broadcast algorithm design far away from trial and worthy of being handled holistically. As reviewed in Sect. 4.2, no existing work, to the best of our knowledge, can solve Problem 4.1 with all requirements satisfied.

## 4.1.2  Summary of Contributions

To fill this void, this chapter systematically addresses the multi-channel broadcast problem from the perspectives of theoretical framework and algorithm design. Specifically, the main contributions of this chapter can be articulated as follows:

- *Theoretical framework*. We establish a theoretical framework on multi-channel broadcast and derive the performance bound of any multi-channel broadcast algorithm. The theoretical results not only shed light on the structure of Problem 4.1, but also direct the design of a reliable and efficient broadcast algorithm.
- *Algorithm design*. With the guidance of the theoretical results, we further design a suite of two multi-channel broadcast (MCB) algorithms, with the latter decreasing the worst-case broadcast delay of the former by up to half via enhancing the duty cycle granularity, and prove they both guarantee broadcast delivery with order-minimal worst-case delay in the asynchronous and heterogeneous environment both theoretically and experimentally.

## 4.2  Related Work

Broadcast is one of the most fundamental services in wireless communications. It facilitates sensor nodes to successfully transmit data to the sink. As during networking configuration, control messages may be broadcast from the sink to all sensor nodes. For data collection, query or interest messages may be broadcasted in the whole network. Hence, implementing an effective broadcast protocol is critical to the overall performance of WBSNs. Moreover, the sink and sensor nodes can operate on multiple channels as specified in IEEE 802.15.6 standard [8]. However, the multi-channel broadcast has not yet been studied in the context of duty-cycling environment. To the best of our knowledge, a number of algorithms have been proposed to solve broadcast problem in WSNs and ad hoc networks but without involving both heterogeneous duty cycles and multiple channels simultaneously.

In duty-cycling WBSNs, sensor nodes often alternative between active and sleep states to reduce the energy consumption. Thus, the sensor nodes with low duty cycles will have a much longer lifetime. As the sink and sensor nodes may have heterogeneous duty cycles based on their individual applications, it may be impossible to wake up all nodes for broadcast through global synchronization. A broadcast protocol accommodating the schedules of the sink and sensor nodes is thus expected for WBSNs. As a representative of the groundbreaking work, the authors in [9] have verified that the conventional broadcast approach may suffer from severe performance degradation under low duty cycles. They could easily fail to wake up at the same time slot. Therefore, the authors have remodeled the duty-cycling broadcast problem in sensor networks, seeking a balance between efficiency and latency with coverage guarantees in [9]. And the problem can be translated into a graph equivalence to resolve by a centralized optimal algorithm.

In [10, 11], Jiao et al. have presented a minimum latency broadcast schedule which aims to find a collision-free scheduling for broadcast with the minimum latency. In duty cycled multi-hop wireless networks, the broadcast schedule problem for both the one-to-all and all-to-all has been proved to be NP-hardness. The authors present one novel approximation algorithm which can provide a broadcast scheduling with a constant approximation ratio.

For low duty-cycling wireless networks, to broadcast a packet, the sink has to transmit the same message multiple times as the sensor nodes do not wake up at the same time. In order to reduce redundancy in transmission while achieving fast dissemination, Guo et al. have proposed a probabilistic flooding scheme to deal with the duty-cycling broadcast problem based on the delay distribution of next-hop receivers in [12]. The key idea of this work lies in the forwarding decision making where a node forwards a packet with a higher probability if the packet arrives opportunistically earlier. Moreover, to alleviate the hidden terminal problems without the RTS and CTS overhead, the authors also propose a forwarder selection method which allows the nodes with good link quality to overhear each other.

The authors in [13] mainly investigate the problem of how to achieve energy-efficient broadcast with minimum latency for low duty cycle WSNs. A novel broadcasting communication model which fully exploits the spatiotemporal locality of broadcasting to reduce the total number of broadcasting message transmissions is proposed to achieve optimal latency and high energy efficiency of broadcasting. The key novelty is to allow nodes to adjust their wake-up schedules to overhear forwarding messages sent by their neighbors. Some nodes which are not on latency-critical paths may postpone their wake-up slots to receive the broadcasting message. Then an approximate algorithm achieving a polylogarithmic approximation ratio is derived to essentially avoid the redundant transmissions and reduce the collision probability as much as possible. Nevertheless, in all the work above, each node needs to know its neighbor working scheduling information a priori, which is unrealistic and does not differ the duty-cycling broadcast from the traditional one materially. In addition, none of them take multi-channel setting into consideration.

The aforementioned works are studied based on single-channel environment. However, to alleviate bandwidth limitations and improve throughput and reliability in wireless communications, the sink and sensor nodes are allowed to operate on multiple frequency channels. Multi-channel communication pattern provides an additional dimension to the broadcast problem. In recent years, a number of algorithms have been proposed to solve the multi-channel broadcast problem in WSNs and ad hoc networks.

In traditional ad hoc networks, broadcast messages are delivered via a common channel which can be heard by all nodes, since the spectrum availability is uniform. However, in cognitive radio ad hoc networks, different unlicensed users may acquire different available channel sets. This non-uniform spectrum availability imposes special design challenges for broadcasting in cognitive radio ad hoc networks. In [14], Song and Xie have proposed a fully distributed broadcast scheme that constructs the broadcasting sequences for both sender and receiver without the requirement of a common control channel, the global network topology, the spectrum availability information of other users, and the clock synchronization. By intelligently downsizing the original available channel set and designing the broadcasting sequences and scheduling schemes, the broadcast protocol can provide very high successful broadcast ratio and eliminate broadcast collisions while achieving the shortest average broadcast delay.

In [15], Dabideen et al. have presented a simplicial-complex-based broadcast algorithm to reduce the transmission times by grouping the neighbors with at least one same channel. The complex activation broadcasting algorithm captures naturally occurring groups and builds a tree that exploits them in real-world multi-channel multi-radio networks.

For efficient broadcast in multi-channel networks, Lim et al. [16] have proposed a novel scheme where a new signal processing mechanism for WLAN to decode the rendezvous information transmitted on the sub-channels which falls in the overlapped band of adjacent channels between the sender and the receiver is devised. The overlapped band which is the frequency range that partially overlapped channels share within their channel boundaries is leveraged. Specifically, a sender advertises the rendezvous channel through the overlapped band of adjacent channels, while the broadcast message is done on the rendezvous channel. However, this work has high requirement on the capability of nodes, which goes against the lightweight nature of WBSNs. Moreover, it cannot satisfy asynchronous clocks and asymmetrical channel perceptions.

Chen et al. have addressed the multi-channel broadcast problem in one-hop infrastructure based cognitive radio networks by exploiting Langford Paring and Skolem Sequence to design the channel hopping sequences, respectively, in [17, 18]. Every broadcast radio at the base station selectively transmits over a number of channels via a channel hopping sequence which is generated using a mathematical construct Langford Paring and Skolem Sequence to guarantee successful broadcast delivery. The channel hopping sequence can satisfy that the base station is free to customize the number of broadcast channels; meanwhile, the induced broadcast delay can be significantly reduced given the number of broadcast channels. However, neither of them can be used in duty-cycling WBSNs where the mathematical properties of Langford Paring and Skolem Sequence cannot be satisfied.

In summary, no existing work has been done on the broadcast problem with the consideration of two dimensions of multi-channel and duty cycle despite their considerable applications in practical networks. In order to bridge this gap, we will design a reliable multi-channel wake-up schedule to addressing the multi-channel broadcast problem in duty-cycling WBSNs from the perspectives of theoretical framework and algorithm design.

## 4.3   Problem Formulation

### 4.3.1   System Model

We consider a time-slotted (but not synchronized) energy-constraint duty-cycling WBSN with one sink and a set $\mathcal{R}$ of $R$ sensor nodes of a single radio interface operating on $N$ frequent channels in a channel set $\mathcal{N}$, i.e., $N \triangleq |\mathcal{N}|$. We assume that sensor node $a$ has the smallest duty cycle in $\mathcal{R}$. In multi-channel environment, the sink and each node wake up periodically and can switch across different channels. In this chapter, we first analyze the symmetrical channel perceptions and then extend to the asymmetrical case. Given such a WBSN, the objective of this chapter is to design efficient deterministic broadcast algorithms.

The main design challenges needed to address in the algorithm design are summarized as follows:

- *Lack of clock synchronization*: Due to the resource constraint, it is extremely difficult to maintain tight synchronization, thus the clocks between the sink and sensor nodes may drift away from each other by an arbitrary amount of time, which may lead to the broadcast failure.
- *Asymmetric duty cycles*: The duty cycles of the sink and the nodes are typically asymmetric, depending on their independent energy constraint and individual applications. Multi-channel broadcast algorithm in duty-cycling WBSNs should ensure that the sink and each node can wake up in a same slot at least regardless of their duty cycles.
- *Broadcast via channel hopping*: To implement the multi-channel broadcast, the sink and each node can hop across multiple channels to deliver or receive the broadcast message. The message can be delivered successfully from the sink to one node if they hop to the same channel in the same time slot. Therefore, we need to design the channel hopping sequence to define the order with which the sink or a node visit the broadcast channel set.

In the following, we formally define the multi-channel hopping schedule for an arbitrary node $u$.

**Definition 4.1 (Channel Hopping Schedule)** The channel hopping schedule of a node $u$ is defined as a sequence $x_u \triangleq \{x_u^t\}_{1 \leq t \leq T_u}$, where $T_u$ is the period of the sequence, and

$$
x_u^t = \begin{cases} 0, & u \text{ sleeps in slot } t \\ h \in \mathcal{N}, & u \text{ wakes up, operating on channel } h. \end{cases}
$$

Thus, we can represent the channel hopping sequence for node $u$ as

$$x_u = \{x_u^1, x_u^2, \ldots, x_u^i, \ldots, x_u^{T_u}\},$$

where $x_u^t \in [0, N]$. If $x_u^i = x_u^{i+1}$, $\forall i \in [1, T_u - 1]$, the node $u$ stays on the same channel and does not hop.

Consider that the sink $s$ intends to broadcast messages to each of the sensor nodes named $u$ without loss of generality. Given two channel hopping sequences of $x_u$ and $x_s$ whose periods are $T_u$ and $T_s$, respectively, if there exists $t \in [1, T_u T_s]$ such that $x_u^t = x_s^t = h$, where $h \in [1, N]$, we say that $s$ can deliver a message to $u$ in the $t$-th time slot on broadcast channel $h$. The $t$-th time slot is called a *broadcast delivery slot* and channel $h$ is called a *broadcast delivery channel* between $u$ and $s$.

Let $\mathcal{T}(x_u, x_s)$ denote the *set of broadcast delivery slots* between two channel hopping sequences $x_u$ and $x_s$, and $|\mathcal{T}(x_u, x_s)| \in [1, T_u T_s]$. The element of $\mathcal{T}(x_u, x_s)$ reflects time slot number in which successful broadcast delivery occurs within a period.

Given $N$ broadcast channels, let $\mathcal{C}(x_u, x_s)$ denote the *set of broadcast delivery channels* between two channel hopping sequences $x_u$ and $x_s$. The cardinality of $\mathcal{C}(x_u, x_s)$ denotes the number of broadcast delivery channels, i.e., $|\mathcal{C}(x_u, x_s)| \in [0, N]$, which measures the broadcast diversity, i.e., the number of channels in which the successful broadcast delivery occurs.

**Definition 4.2 (Duty Cycle)** The duty cycle of a node $u$, denoted by $\delta_u$, is defined as the percentage of active time slots per period of the channel hopping schedule $x_u$. Formally, $\delta_u$ is expressed as

$$\delta_u \triangleq \frac{|t \in [1, T_u] : x_u^t \neq 0|}{T_u}.$$

The reciprocal of $\delta_u$ is denoted by $d_u$.

**Definition 4.3 (Clock Drift)** We apply *cyclic rotation* to model the situation where the clocks of different nodes are not synchronized. Specifically, given a channel hopping schedule $x_u$, we denote $x_u(k)$ a cyclic rotation of $x_u$ by $k$ slots, thus

$$x_u(k) = \{r_u^t\}_{1 \leq t \leq T_u},$$

where $r_u^t = x_u^{(t+k) \bmod T_u}$. For example, given $x_u = \{0, 1, 2\}$, where $T_u = 3$, $x_u(2) = x_u(-1) = \{2, 0, 1\}$.

In order to guarantee successful broadcast delivery, the channel hopping sequences of $x_u$ and $x_s$ must satisfy that the number of broadcast delivery channels is greater than or equal to 1 for all possible clock drifts, i.e., $|\mathcal{C}(x_u(k), x_s(l))| \geq 1$, $\forall k, l \in \mathbb{Z}$.

### 4.3.2  Performance Metrics

Here, given a multi-channel broadcast algorithm for WBSNs, we introduce the following metrics for evaluating its performance:

- **Broadcast delay**: To quantify the broadcast delay (BD), we use the worst-case broadcast delay that is the upper bound of the time (in number of slots) needed by the sink to broadcast control information to an arbitrary sensor node for the first time regardless of their duty cycles for all possible clock drifts, i.e.,

$$\max_{u \in \mathcal{R}, \forall \delta_u, \delta_s, \forall k, l \in \mathbb{Z}} (\min \mathcal{T}(\mathrm{x}_u(k), \mathrm{x}_s(l))).$$

- **Broadcast diversity**: The broadcast diversity characterizes the capability of a multi-channel broadcast algorithm of delivering broadcast message regardless of its operational channel, which measures the lower bound of broadcast delivery channel set size between the sink and an arbitrary sensor node with any duty cycle and clock drift. The broadcast diversity is thus expressed as

$$\mathrm{DIV} = \min_{\forall \delta_u, \delta_s, \forall k, l \in \mathbb{Z}} |\mathcal{C}(\mathrm{x}_u(k), \mathrm{x}_s(l))|.$$

We say that a multi-channel broadcast algorithm achieves *full* broadcast diversity if the broadcast delivery between the sink and an arbitrary sensor node is guaranteed on *every* common channel they can access, i.e., DIV=$N$, where $N$ is the number of the common channels.

- **Broadcast delay with full diversity**: Full diversity implies the robustness of a multi-channel broadcast algorithm. Thereby, we further define the third metric *broadcast delay with full diversity* (BD-FD) as the upper bound of the worst-case delay before the full broadcast diversity is achieved at the first time, which is given by

$$\max_{u \in \mathcal{R}, \forall \delta_u, \delta_s, \forall k, l \in \mathbb{Z}} (\min \mathcal{T}(\mathrm{x}_u(k), \mathrm{x}_s(l)))$$

$$\text{subject to} \quad \mathrm{DIV} = N.$$

Note that the BD-FD degenerates to the BD in single-channel case. In this chapter, we will analyze the BD in single-channel case and the BD-FD in multi-channel case.

### 4.3.3  Optimal Problem

In order to ensure the reliable broadcast delivery between the sink and any sensor node in a WBSN, we would ideally want a multi-channel broadcast algorithm to achieve full broadcast diversity. Therefore, our objective is to devise channel hopping sequences for the sink and any sensor node that not only guarantee the successful broadcast delivery but also have the minimum broadcast delay and the maximum broadcast diversity for any duty cycle pair $(\delta_u, \delta_s)$, any initial time offset $t_u^0$ and $t_s^0$ (i.e., any clock drifts), and any channel set $\mathcal{N}$. The optimal multi-channel broadcast problem can be formulated as follows:

$$
\begin{aligned}
\text{minimize} \quad & \max_{u \in \mathcal{R}} (\min \mathcal{T}(x_u(k), x_s(l))) \\
\text{s. t.:} \quad & \min |\mathcal{C}(x_u(k), x_s(l))| = N \\
& \forall t_u^0 \in [1, T_u], t_s^0 \in [1, T_s], \forall \delta_u, \delta_s, \exists t \le T \\
& \text{such that } x_u^t(t_u^0) = x_s^t(t_s^0) = h, \forall h \in \mathcal{N}.
\end{aligned}
\tag{4.1}
$$

To streamline this chapter, in what follows, we first establish a theoretical performance bound of any multi-channel broadcast algorithm and then design individual channel hopping sequences for the sink and sensor nodes.

## 4.4   Multi-Channel Broadcast Delay Bound

In this section, we derive the generalized lower bound of the solution to the optimal problem (4.1).

**Theorem 4.1** *For any multi-channel broadcast algorithm solving the optimal problem (4.1), the BD-FD, denoted by L, is lower-bounded by $N^2 d_a d_s$ where s is the sink and a is the sensor node with the smallest duty cycle in $\mathcal{R}$ and $d_a = \frac{1}{\delta_a}$ and $d_s = \frac{1}{\delta_s}$.*

*Proof* For any sensor node $u$ and the sink $s$, their channel hopping sequences are denoted as $x_u$ and $x_s$ with the periods of $T_u$ and $T_s$, respectively. Because the channel hopping schedules of $u$ and $s$ repeat every $T_u T_s$ time slots regardless of the clock drifts, if the successful broadcast delivery can occur with full diversity regardless of the clock drifts, the worst-case BD-FD $L$ should be upper-bounded by $T_u T_s$.

Without loss of generality, we fix $x_u$ and cyclically rotate $x_s$ by $l$ slots with $l = 0, 1, \ldots, T_u T_s - 1$. Since the BD-FD is the maximum broadcast delay with full diversity for any initial clock offsets of $u$ and $s$, there must exist at least $N$ broadcast delivery slots among $L$ slots when both $u$ and $s$ wake up and hop to the same channel. Thus, the minimal number of broadcast delivery slots are $\frac{N T_u T_s}{L}$ within consecutive $T_u T_s$ slots. Let $S$ denote the total number of accumulated broadcast delivery slots within consecutive $T_u T_s$ slots between $x_u$ and $x_s(l)$ as $l$ is incremented from 0 to $T_u T_s - 1$, we have

$$
S \ge \frac{N(T_u T_s)^2}{L}.
\tag{4.2}
$$

On the other hand, let $n_u^h$ ($n_s^h$, respectively) denote the number of time slots in $x_u$ ($x_s$, respectively) in which $u$ ($s$) wakes up on channel $h$ within consecutive $T_u T_s$ slots. We can express the reciprocals of the duty cycles of $u$ and $s$ as

$$d_u = \frac{T_u T_s}{\sum_{h \in \mathcal{N}} n_u^h}, \quad d_s = \frac{T_u T_s}{\sum_{h \in \mathcal{N}} n_s^h}.$$

After some algebraic operations, we obtain

$$T_u T_s = \sum_{h \in \mathcal{N}} d_u n_u^h = \sum_{h \in \mathcal{N}} d_s n_s^h = \sum_{h \in \mathcal{N}} \frac{d_u n_u^h + d_s n_s^h}{2}. \qquad (4.3)$$

Since $x_u$ and $x_s(l)$ achieve full diversity, for any channel $h$, the total accumulated number of broadcast deliveries between $x_u$ and $x_s(l)$ with $l$ incremented from 0 to $T_u T_s - 1$, in which the broadcast channel is $h$, is $S = \sum_{h \in \mathcal{N}} n_u^h n_s^h$. For $d_u n_u^h d_s n_s^h \leq \left( \frac{d_u n_u^h + d_s n_s^h}{2} \right)^2$, it follows from Eq. (4.3) that

$$S = \sum_{h \in \mathcal{N}} n_u^h n_s^h = \frac{\sum_{h \in \mathcal{N}} d_u n_u^h \cdot d_s n_s^h}{d_u d_s} \leq \frac{(T_u T_s)^2}{d_u d_s N}.$$

It then follows from Eq. (4.2) that $\frac{N(T_u T_s)^2}{L} \leq \frac{(T_u T_v)^2}{d_u d_s N}$, which leads to $L \geq N^2 d_u d_s$. Finally, due to $\delta_a = \min_{u \in \mathcal{R}}(\delta_u)$, it should thus hold that $L \geq N^2 d_a d_s$.    $\square$

Theorem 4.1 implies that the performance of any multi-channel broadcast algorithm is determined by the sink and the sensor node with the smallest duty cycle. As further explained in the following remark, we can guarantee the successful broadcast delivery from the sink $s$ to all sensor nodes if the delivery can be achieved between $s$ and $a$ of the smallest duty cycle. Therefore, we focus on the analysis between $s$ and $a$ in what follows. Note that the properties of $a$ in the rest of this chapter also hold for the other sensor nodes.

*Remark* For a WBSN with one sink $s$ and $R$ sensor nodes operating on $N$ broadcast channels, the worst-case BD-FD happens on the broadcast from the sink to the node $a$ of the smallest duty cycle for any multi-channel broadcast algorithm, which is asymptotically $L \simeq O(N^2 d^2)$ when $d_s \simeq d_a \simeq O(d)$.

Given the performance bound of any multi-channel broadcast algorithm, in the following, we design the broadcast algorithms both on single-channel case and multi-channel case, which are optimal in magnitude.

## 4.5  MCB: Single-Channel Case

### 4.5.1  Technical Background

**The Chinese Remainder Theorem (CRT)** Suppose $m_1, \ldots, m_k$ are positive integers that are pairwise co-prime. Then, for any given sequence of integers $b_1, \ldots, b_k$, there exists an integer $x$ solving the following system of simultaneous congruences:

$$\begin{cases} t \equiv b_1 & (\text{mod } m_1) \\ t \equiv b_2 & (\text{mod } m_2) \\ \quad \vdots \\ t \equiv b_k & (\text{mod } m_k). \end{cases}$$

Furthermore, any two solutions of this system are congruent modulo the product $M = \prod_{i=1}^{k} m_i$. Hence, there is a unique (nonnegative) solution less than $M$. The detailed proof can refer to [19].

In the single-channel case, the channel hopping schedule degenerates to a binary sequence whose period is determined by the node's duty cycle. For two distinct nodes $u$ and $v$ with sets of integers $D_u = \{d_1^u, d_2^u, \ldots, d_{|D_u|}^u\}$ and $D_v = \{d_1^v, d_2^v, \ldots, d_{|D_v|}^v\}$, respectively, if there exits an integer in $D_u$ that is co-prime to an integer in $D_v$, i.e., $\exists d_{i_0}^u \in D_u$ and $\exists d_{j_0}^v \in D_v$, such that $d_{i_0}^u$ and $d_{j_0}^v$ are co-prime, then the successful broadcast delivery can be guaranteed between $u$ and $v$ by the CRT. Correspondingly, the wake-up sequence $x_u \triangleq \{x_u^t\}_{1 \leq t \leq T_u}$ of node $u$ under this co-primality is

$$x_u^t = \begin{cases} 1 & t \text{ is divisible by some } d_i^u \in D_u, \\ 0 & \text{otherwise.} \end{cases}$$

The period length is $T_u = \text{lcm}(d_1^u, d_2^u, \ldots, d_{|D_u|}^u)$ and its duty cycle $\delta_u$ is

$$\delta_u = \sum_{1 \leq i_1 \leq |D_u|} \frac{1}{d_{i_1}^u} - \sum_{1 \leq i_1 < i_2 \leq |D_u|} \frac{1}{\text{lcm}(d_{i_1}^u, d_{i_2}^u)} \cdots$$
$$+ (-1)^{|D_u|+1} \frac{1}{\text{lcm}(d_1^u, d_2^u, \ldots, d_{|D_u|}^u)}.$$

The same results still hold for node $v$. Moreover, we can obtain the following theorem from the CRT.

**Theorem 4.2** *The broadcast delivery between any pair of nodes $u$ and $v$ can be guaranteed for any amount of clock drifts if their associated integer sets satisfy the* *co-primality. That is, if $d_u$ and $d_v$ are co-prime to each other, there exactly exists a solution $t \equiv t_d$ (mod $d_u d_v$) in every period $d = d_u d_v$ such that $x_u^{t_d} = x_v^{t_d} (\delta_{uv}) = 1$, $\forall \delta_{uv} \in \mathbb{Z}$, for the following congruence system:*

$$\begin{cases} t \equiv 0 & (\text{mod } d_u) \\ t + \delta_{uv} \equiv 0 & (\text{mod } d_v), \end{cases}$$

*where $\delta_{uv}$ is the clock drift between $u$ and $v$.*

*And the broadcast delay is bounded by the product of the two smallest co-prime numbers, one from each set, i.e.:*

$$\min_{gcd(d_i^u, d_j^v)=1, 1 \leq i \leq D_u, 1 \leq j \leq D_v} \{d_i^u \cdot d_j^v\}.$$

This theorem states that if $t_d \in [1, d_u d_v]$ is such a solution, then an integer $t$ satisfies the congruences if and only if $t$ is of the form $t = t_d + kd$ for $k = 1, 2, \ldots$.

### 4.5.2  Algorithm Design

Motivated by the CRT and Theorem 4.2, given the desired duty cycles of the sink and any sensor node in WBSNs, if their designed reciprocals of duty cycles are co-prime to each other, the successful broadcast delivery between them is guaranteed for any amount of clock drifts. Thus, we devise the following MCB wake-up schedules for the sink and node $a$ in single-channel case, respectively.

To be precise, the wake-up schedule for the sink $s$ with duty cycle $\delta_s = \frac{1}{d_s}$ can be generated as:

$$x_s^t = \begin{cases} 1 & t \text{ is divisible by } p_s, \\ 0 & \text{otherwise,} \end{cases}$$

where $p_s = 2^k$ and $k = \lceil \log_2 d_s \rceil$.

Correspondingly, for node $a$ with the smallest duty cycle $\delta_a = \frac{1}{d_a}$ in $\mathcal{R}$ generates its wake-up schedule based on

$$x_a^t = \begin{cases} 1 & t \text{ is divisible by } p_a, \\ 0 & \text{otherwise,} \end{cases}$$

where $p_a$ is the smallest odd integer which minimizes $|p_a - d_a|$.

Therefore, the broadcast delivery between $s$ and $a$ occurs successfully regardless of their clock drifts, as the $p_s$ and $p_a$ are co-prime following from the CRT and

Theorem 4.2, which will be explained in Theorem 4.3. Example 4.1 illustrates the MCB algorithm in single-channel case.

*Example 4.1* Consider the sink $s$ and node $a$ with duty cycles $\delta_s = \frac{1}{3}$ and $\delta_a = \frac{1}{6}$, respectively, we can derive that $p_s = 4$ and $p_a = 7$ under the designed MCB wake-up schedules. Using the time of $s$ as a reference, if there is a clock drift $\delta_{sa} = 2$, $s$ wakes up in slots $4k$, i.e., $4, 8, 12, \ldots$, and $a$ wakes up in slots $7k + 2$, i.e., $9, 16, 23, \ldots$, as illustrated in Fig. 4.1. The broadcast delivery happens in slot $16 + 28k$, $k = 1, 2, 3, \ldots$ between $s$ and $a$.

### 4.5.3 Duty Cycle Granularity

Here we discuss the granularity of the MCB in matching any desired duty cycle in practical applications. Consider the desired duty cycle of node $u$ is $\delta_u$ and its actual value $\hat{\delta_u}$, the relative error $\epsilon(\delta_u)$ between $\delta_u$ and $\hat{\delta_u}$ is defined by

$$\epsilon(\delta_u) = \frac{|\hat{\delta_u} - \delta_u|}{\delta_u}.$$

Following the wake-up schedule in MCB, the actual duty cycle of the sink $s$ is $\hat{\delta_s} = \frac{1}{2^k}$, while the required one is $\delta_s = \frac{1}{d_s}$. According to the definition of the relative error, we have

$$\epsilon(\delta_s) = \frac{|\hat{\delta_s} - \delta_s|}{\delta_s} = \left| \frac{1}{2^{\lceil \log_2 d_s \rceil}} - \frac{1}{d_s} \right| / \frac{1}{d_s} < \frac{1}{2}. \tag{4.4}$$

Similarly, we can also derive the relative error of node $a$ between $\hat{\delta_a}$ and $\delta_a$ as

$$\epsilon(\delta_a) = \left| \frac{1}{p_a} - \frac{1}{d_a} \right| / \frac{1}{d_a} \le \frac{1}{d_a - 1}. \tag{4.5}$$

As shown in Eq. (4.5), the relative error of node $a$ decreases with the decline of the desired duty cycle $\delta_a$. In practical applications of WBSNs, $\delta_a$ is typically very low, thus $\epsilon(\delta_a)$ is small enough. However, the relative error $\epsilon(\delta_s)$ is not very

| Slot index | 1 | 2 | 3 | 4 | 5 | 6 | 7 | 8 | 9 | 10 | 11 | 12 | 13 | 14 | 15 | 16 | 17 | 18 | ... |
|---|---|---|---|---|---|---|---|---|---|---|---|---|---|---|---|---|---|---|---|
| Sink s: | 0 | 0 | 0 | 1 | 0 | 0 | 0 | 1 | 0 | 0 | 0 | 1 | 0 | 0 | 0 | 1 | 0 | 0 | ... |
| Node a: | 0 | 0 | 0 | 0 | 0 | 0 | 0 | 0 | 1 | 0 | 0 | 0 | 0 | 0 | 0 | 1 | 0 | 0 | ... |

**Fig. 4.1** MCB in single-channel case: $d_s = 3$, $d_a = 6$

stringent to approach the required duty cycle as in Eq. (4.4). In order to improve the granularity of the sink, we will propose an improved MCB design in Sect. 4.7.

### 4.5.4  Broadcast Delay

In the single-channel case, only the first performance metric is applicable. By the CRT and Theorem 4.2, we derive and state the broadcast delay of MCB in the single-channel case in the worst case in the following Theorem 4.3.

**Theorem 4.3** *Given the duty cycles of the sink $\frac{1}{d_s}$ and node a $\frac{1}{d_a}$, as $p_s$ and $p_a$ are co-prime with each other, the successful broadcast delivery is ensured to occur within at most $p_s p_a$ time slots for any amount of clock drifts.*

*Proof* Based on the algorithm design of MCB in single-channel, the wake-up period $p_s$ of the sink $s$ is a power-multiple of 2, and the wake-up period $p_a$ of node $a$ is an odd integer. It thus holds that $p_s$ is co-prime with $p_a$. It follows from the CRT and Theorem 4.2 that broadcast delivery occurs between $s$ and $a$ of the smallest duty cycle within at most $p_s p_a$ slots, regardless of their clock offset.    □

## 4.6  MCB: Multi-Channel Case

In this section, we proceed to develop MCB for the multi-channel case which achieves the full diversity within the order-minimum BD-FD.

### 4.6.1  Motivation and Algorithm Design

Robust broadcast algorithm in multi-channel case performs differently from that in single-channel case, as it needs to ensure that the sink and nodes not only wake up in the same slot but also hop to the same channel and to achieve the full diversity. Thus, consider a WBSN of $N$ channels, where the sink and nodes can hop across all the $N$ channels based on their individual duty cycles, respectively, our objective is to develop multi-channel hopping schedules for the sink and nodes which guarantee the successful broadcast delivery with full diversity within the bounded broadcast delay.

Based on the wake-up schedules in single-channel case in Sect. 4.5.2 and following from the CRT and Theorem 4.2, the broadcast delivery with full diversity can be guaranteed if and only if the intervals of time slots when the sink and sensor nodes hop to the same channel are co-prime with each other. Motivated by this observation, we devise the following MCB channel hopping schedules for the sink and all sensor nodes in multi-channel case, respectively, and will explain the design rationale in Theorem 4.4.

Specifically, given $N$ broadcast channels, denote by $q_s$ the period of channel polling for the sink $s$ in active slots and by $m$ the smallest integer satisfying $2^m \geq N$, we then set $q_s = 2^m$ and construct the channel hopping sequence of $s$ as

$$
x_s^t = \begin{cases} h_i & t - ip_s \text{ is divisible by } p_s q_s, 0 < i \leq N, \\ h_r & t - ip_s \text{ is divisible by } p_s q_s, N < i \leq q_s, \\ 0 & \text{otherwise,} \end{cases} \qquad (4.6)
$$

where $h_r$ denotes a channel randomly selected in $[1, N]$. It can be noted that the whole period of the channel hopping sequence $x_s$ is $p_s q_s$.

Similarly, let $q_a$ denote the period of channel polling for node $a$ in active slots, we set it to the smallest odd integer which is not smaller than $N$. Correspondingly, the channel hopping sequence of $a$ is generated as:

$$
x_a^t = \begin{cases} h_i & t - ip_a \text{ is divisible by } p_a q_a, 0 < i \leq N, \\ h_r & t - ip_a \text{ is divisible by } p_a q_a, N < i \leq q_a, \\ 0 & \text{otherwise,} \end{cases} \qquad (4.7)
$$

and the period of $x_a$ is $p_a q_a$. Example 4.2 illustrates the channel hopping sequences for $s$ and $a$.

*Example 4.2* Consider the sink $s$ and node $a$ with duty cycles $\delta_s = \frac{1}{3}$ and $\delta_a = \frac{1}{6}$, respectively, operating on three common channels (i.e., $N = 3$). Under the above MCB channel hopping schedules, we can derive that $p_s = 4$, $q_s = 4$, $p_a = 7$, and $q_a = 3$. Using the time of $s$ as a reference, $s$ wakes up on channel $h_1$ in slots $4 + 16k$, i.e., $4, 20, 36, \ldots$, on channel $h_2$ in slots $8 + 16k$, i.e., $8, 24, 40, \ldots$, and on channel $h_3$ in slots $12 + 16k$, i.e., $12, 28, 44, \ldots$. It can be noted that $s$ wakes up and randomly hops to one channel in the slots $16 + 16k$, $k = 0, 1, 2, 3, \ldots$. Similarly, $a$ wakes up on channel $h_1$ in slots $7 + 21k$, on channel $h_2$ in slots $14 + 21k$, and on channel $h_3$ in slots $21 + 21k$, $k = 0, 1, 2, 3, \ldots$, as illustrated in Fig. 4.2a. The first

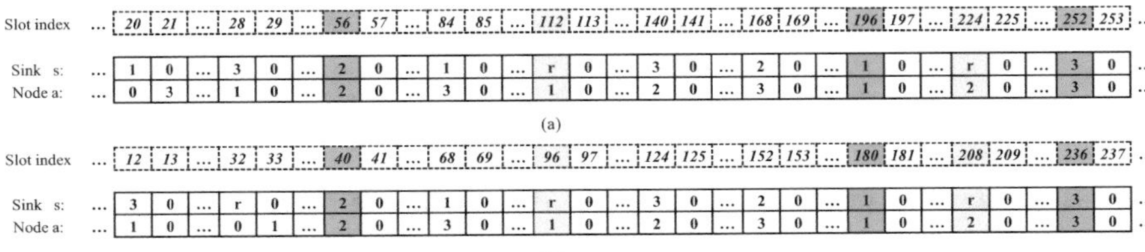

| Slot index | ... | 20 | 21 | ... | 28 | 29 | ... | 56 | 57 | ... | 84 | 85 | ... | 112 | 113 | ... | 140 | 141 | ... | 168 | 169 | ... | 196 | 197 | ... | 224 | 225 | ... | 252 | 253 | ... |
|---|---|---|---|---|---|---|---|---|---|---|---|---|---|---|---|---|---|---|---|---|---|---|---|---|---|---|---|---|---|---|---|
| Sink s: | ... | 1 | 0 | ... | 3 | 0 | ... | 2 | 0 | ... | 1 | 0 | ... | r | 0 | ... | 3 | 0 | ... | 2 | 0 | ... | 1 | 0 | ... | r | 0 | ... | 3 | 0 | ... |
| Node a: | ... | 0 | 3 | ... | 1 | 0 | ... | 2 | 0 | ... | 3 | 0 | ... | 1 | 0 | ... | 2 | 0 | ... | 3 | 0 | ... | 1 | 0 | ... | 2 | 0 | ... | 3 | 0 | ... |

(a)

| Slot index | ... | 12 | 13 | ... | 32 | 33 | ... | 40 | 41 | ... | 68 | 69 | ... | 96 | 97 | ... | 124 | 125 | ... | 152 | 153 | ... | 180 | 181 | ... | 208 | 209 | ... | 236 | 237 | ... |
|---|---|---|---|---|---|---|---|---|---|---|---|---|---|---|---|---|---|---|---|---|---|---|---|---|---|---|---|---|---|---|---|
| Sink s: | ... | 3 | 0 | ... | r | 0 | ... | 2 | 0 | ... | 1 | 0 | ... | r | 0 | ... | 3 | 0 | ... | 2 | 0 | ... | 1 | 0 | ... | r | 0 | ... | 3 | 0 | ... |
| Node a: | ... | 1 | 0 | ... | 0 | 1 | ... | 2 | 0 | ... | 3 | 0 | ... | 1 | 0 | ... | 2 | 0 | ... | 3 | 0 | ... | 1 | 0 | ... | 2 | 0 | ... | 3 | 0 | ... |

(b)

**Fig. 4.2** MCB in multi-channel case: $d_s = 3$, $d_a = 6$. (**a**) Without clock drift. (**b**) Node a drifts by 5 time slots to the right

successful broadcast delivery happens at the 56th slot, and the broadcast delivery with full diversity achieves at the 252nd slot between $s$ and $a$. Correspondingly, if there exists a clock drift offset, such as $\delta_{sa} = 5$, the broadcast delivery firstly occurs at the 40th slot, and the broadcast delivery with full diversity can also be ensured at the 236th slot between $s$ and $a$ as shown in Fig. 4.2b. Note that the entries with value $r$ indicate a random number in $[1, N]$, thus the broadcast delivery may also occur in the 112nd and 234th slots as shown in Fig. 4.2a.

## 4.6.2   Broadcast Delay

In multi-channel case, the second metric on broadcast diversity and third metric on BD-FD are applicable. By the CRT and Theorem 4.2, we can derive that MCB can achieve full diversity within bounded broadcast delay as shown in the following Theorem 4.4.

**Theorem 4.4** *Given the number of broadcast channels $N$ in a WBSN and the required full diversity, i.e., DIV= $N$, for $\forall u \in \mathcal{R}$. If $\frac{1}{d_s}$ and $\frac{1}{d_a}$ are the duty cycles of the sink $s$ and the node $a$ with the smallest duty cycle, respectively, the BD-FD is equal to $p_s q_s p_a q_a$, regardless of their clock drifts. Asymptotically, when $q_s \simeq q_a \simeq O(N)$, BD-FD $\simeq O(N^2 p_s p_a)$.*

*Proof* Following the algorithm design of MCB in multi-channel case, the period of the channel hopping sequence of the sink $x_s$ is $p_s q_s = 2^{k+m}$ which is an even integer, and the period of $x_a$ is $p_a q_a$ which is an odd integer. It is well-known that the even integer and odd integer are co-prime. It then follows from the CRT and Theorem 4.2 that there exists $t_0 < p_s q_s p_a q_a$ such that $x_s^{t_0}(t_s^0) = x_a^{t_0}(t_a^0) = h$ for any channel $h$ and it holds that on slots $t_k = t_0 + k p_s q_s p_a q_a$, the broadcast delivery can be ensured to occur between the sink $s$ and node $a$. Therefore, MCB achieves the full diversity within at most $O(N^2 p_s p_a)$ time slots.                    $\square$

The capability of achieving broadcast delivery on every channel within bounded delay significantly improves broadcast communication robustness in wireless environment where channel condition is unpredictable and may vary in both time and space.

## 4.7   An Improved MCB

In this section, we propose an improved MCB to further decrease the broadcast delay in the worst case, and analyze its robustness against asymmetrical channel perception between the sink and sensor nodes, subsequently.

### 4.7.1   An Improved Algorithm

Recall the analysis of duty cycle granularity in Sect. 4.5.3, the relative error of a sensor node $\epsilon(\delta_a)$ is typically very small, as the $p_a$ is the smallest odd integer not smaller than $d_a$ in our design. It is well-known that we can find $p_a$ which is very close to $d_a$ for any $d_a$. However, the relative error of the sink $\epsilon(\delta_s)$ may be up to $\frac{1}{2}$ as shown in Eq. (4.4). The main reason is that we design $p_s$ as a power-multiple of 2 to approximate the desired $d_s$. In the extremely unlucky case where $d_s$ is in the form of $2^n + 1$, we may have $p_s \simeq 2d_s$ when the broadcast delay in the worst case is $p_s p_a \simeq 2d_s d_a$. Similarly, in MCB for multi-channel case, as $q_s$ needs to be a power-multiple of 2, we may also have $q_s \simeq 2N$ in the worst case, thus leading to larger BD-FD, i.e., $p_s q_s p_a q_a \simeq 2N^2 p_s p_a \simeq 4N^2 d_s d_a$.

Motivated by the above observations, we propose an improved MCB to further limit the upper bound of the broadcast delay even in the extremely unlucky case. Specifically, in the improved MCB, given the duty cycle $\delta_s$, the sink $s$ independently set $p_s = 2^{k_1} 3^{k_2}$ with integers $k_1$ and $k_2$ chosen from $[0, \lceil log_2 d_s \rceil]$ and $[0, \lceil log_3 d_s \rceil]$, respectively, such that $p_s - d_s$ is minimized under the constraint $p_s \geq d_s$, i.e.,

$$(k_1, k_2) = \operatorname*{argmin}_{k_1, k_2}(2^{k_1} 3^{k_2} - d_s), \quad \text{s.t.} \quad 2^{k_1} 3^{k_2} \geq d_s.$$

Lemma 4.1 proves that $p_s$ is asymptotically close to $d_s$.

**Lemma 4.1** *For any $\epsilon > 0$, given $d_s$ sufficiently large, there exist $k_1 \in [0, \lceil log_2 d_s \rceil]$ and $k_2 \in [0, \lceil log_3 d_s \rceil]$ so that $p_s = 2^{k_1} 3^{k_2} \geq d_s$ and $p_s - d_s \leq \epsilon$, i.e., $d_s$ can be arbitrarily closely approximated by $q_s$.*

*Proof* We give the proof sketch. We prove the lemma by showing for large enough $d_s$ that there exist $k_1 \in [0, \lceil log_2 d_s \rceil]$ and $k_2 \in [0, \lceil log_3 d_s \rceil]$ such that

$$log_2 d_s \leq k_1 + k_2 log_2 3 < log_2 d_s + \epsilon.$$

This follows from the fact that the fractional parts of $x log_2 3$ for $x \in \mathbb{N}$, i.e., $x log_2 3 - \lfloor x log_2 3 \rfloor$, are dense in $[0, 1]$. In fact, given any $\epsilon > 0$, if we choose nonnegative integers $\{x_i\}$ so that fractional parts of $x log_2 3$ form an $\frac{\epsilon}{2}$ set of $[0, 1]$, then we can choose the appropriate integer $k_2$ and then $k_1$, which is feasible provided that $d_s$ is large enough. □

Similarly, given the number of broadcast channels $N$, the sink $s$ can set $q_s = 2^{m_1} 3^{m_2}$ where $m_1$ and $m_2$ are the integers chosen from $[0, \lceil log_2 N \rceil]$ and $[0, \lceil log_3 N \rceil]$, respectively, so that $q_s - N$ is minimized under the constraint $q_s \geq N$, i.e.,

$$(m_1, m_2) = \operatorname*{argmin}_{m_1, m_2}(2^{m_1} 3^{m_2} - N), \quad \text{s.t.} \quad 2^{m_1} 3^{m_2} \geq N.$$

Correspondingly, following from the CRT and Theorem 4.2, the successful broadcast delivery between the sink $s$ and node $a$ can be guaranteed as long as $p_s q_s$ is co-prime with $p_a q_a$. Therefore, $p_a$ and $q_a$ need to be co-prime to 2 (or 3) and/or 3 (or 2) depending on $k_1, k_2, m_1, m_2$ in the improved MCB. Specifically, given $p_s$ and $q_s$, we can pick $p_a$ and $q_a$ by solving the following optimization problems:

$$\text{obj: } \min |p_a - d_a| \qquad\qquad \text{obj: } \min(q_a - N)$$

$$\text{s.t.: } p_a > 0 \text{ (mod 2 or/and 3)} \qquad \text{s.t.: } q_a \geq N$$

$$q_a > 0 \text{ (mod 2 or/and 3)}.$$

If the system parameters on duty cycle and channel set are given, we can obtain $p_s, q_s$ first, then $p_a, q_a$, and finally the channel hopping sequences as in Eqs. (4.6) and (4.7).

Furthermore, we can conduct the same analysis as the proof of Theorems 4.3 and 4.4 to show that the worst-case broadcast delay of the improved MCB in the single-channel case is $p_s p_a$, decreasing by half the worst-case asymptotic delay of the original algorithm in the extremely unlucky case, while that in the multi-channel case is $p_s q_s p_a q_a$, a quarter of the original broadcast delay in the worst case.

### 4.7.2   Robustness Against Asymmetrical Channel Perception

In previous analysis, we implicitly assume that the sink and sensor nodes have the same channel perception, i.e., they have symmetrical knowledge on $\mathcal{N}$. Next, we relax this assumption to study the asymmetrical scenario where the sink $s$ and sensor nodes have different perceptions on $\mathcal{N}$. For clarity, we, without loss of generality, assume all sensor nodes have the same channel perception and node $a$ has the smallest duty cycle.

Denoted by $\mathcal{N}_s$ and $\mathcal{N}_a$ which are subsets of $\mathcal{N}$ the channel perceptions of $s$ and $a$, respectively. Specifically, the channel perception asymmetry between $s$ and $a$ can be characterized at two levels:

- *Asymmetry on accessible channel set:* They have asymmetrical perceptions on the global channel set $\mathcal{N}$, i.e., $\mathcal{N}_s \neq \mathcal{N}_a$ and $\mathcal{N}_s \cap \mathcal{N}_a \neq \emptyset$.
- *Asymmetry on channel index:* They have asymmetrical perceptions on the channel index, i.e., channel $h \in \mathcal{N}$ is indexed by $h_i$ by $s$ and $h_j$ by $a$ where $h_i \in \mathcal{N}_s$ and $h_j \in \mathcal{N}_a$ but $h_i \neq h_j$.

The channel hopping schedule of $s$ in MCB thus becomes

$$x_s^t = \begin{cases} h_i & t - ip_s \text{ is divisible by } p_s q_s, 0 < i \leq N_s, \\ h_r & t - ip_s \text{ is divisible by } p_s q_s, N_s < i \leq q_s, \\ 0 & \text{otherwise,} \end{cases}$$

where $h_r$ represents a channel randomly picked by $s$ from $[1, N_s]$. Correspondingly, the channel hopping sequence of $a$ becomes

$$x_a^t = \begin{cases} h_i & t - i p_a \text{ is divisible by } p_a q_a, 0 < i \leq N_a, \\ h_r & t - i p_a \text{ is divisible by } p_a q_a, N_a < i \leq q_a, \\ 0 & \text{otherwise,} \end{cases}$$

where $h_r$ denotes a channel randomly selected from $[1, N_a]$.

The following theorem establishes the performance of MCB in such context.

**Theorem 4.5** *MCB under asymmetrical channel perceptions achieves the same BD-FD as under symmetrical channel perceptions, i.e., within at most $O(N_s N_a d_s d_a)$ (specifically, $O(N^2 d^2)$ if $d_s \simeq d_a \simeq O(d)$ and $N_s \simeq N_a \simeq O(N)$) slots, the successful broadcast delivery from the sink $s$ to all sensor nodes occurs on each common channel $h \in \mathcal{N}_s \cap \mathcal{N}_a$.*

*Proof* Since $p_s q_s$ is co-prime with $p_a q_a$ in our original and improved MCB algorithm designs, it thus holds following from CRT that there exists $t_0 < p_s q_s p_a q_a$ such that $x_s^{t_0}(t_s^0) = h_i$ and $x_a^{t_0}(t_b^0) = h_j$ for any channel $h$ indexed as $h_i$ ($h_j$) by $s$ ($a$). Then by the similar analysis as the proof of Theorem 4.4, we can prove the BD-FD to be $O(N_s N_a d_s d_a)$.   □

Theorem 4.5 shows that MCB is robust against asymmetrical channel perceptions, either on the channel set or index. The following Example 4.3 exemplifies the capability of improved MCB against asymmetrical channel perceptions.

*Example 4.3* Consider a WBSN of four broadcast channels (i.e., $N = 4$), the sink $s$ with desired duty cycle $\delta_s = \frac{1}{5}$ can hop across all the four channels, i.e., $N_s = 4$, and node $a$ with required duty cycle $\delta_a = \frac{1}{8}$ can access three channels, i.e., $N_a = 3$. Under the schedules of improved MCB, we can derive that the actual wake-up period of $s$ is $p_s = 6$ as $k_1 = 1, k_2 = 1$, and the actual period of channel hopping is $q_s = 4$ as $m_1 = 2, m_2 = 0$. Correspondingly, we have $p_a = 7$ and $q_a = 5$. Note that the value $r$ denotes a random number in $[1, N]$. For the asymmetry on accessible channel set, the broadcast delivery with full diversity (i.e., $\mathcal{N}_s \cap \mathcal{N}_a = 3$ and the common channels are $h_1, h_2$ and $h_3$) achieves at the 546th slot between $s$ and $a$ as illustrated in Fig. 4.3a. For the asymmetry on channel index, without loss of generality, assume that the channel $h_1$ indexed by $s$ is indexed by $a$ as $h_2$, $h_3$ for $s$ is denoted by $a$ as $h_1$, and $h_4$ for $s$ is indexed as $h_3$ for $a$. In this case, the successful broadcast delivery with full diversity also happens at 336th slot as shown in Fig. 4.3b.

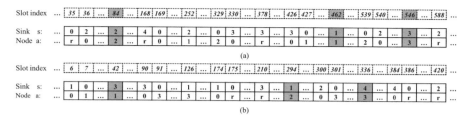

Fig. 4.3 Improved MCB against asymmetrical channel perceptions. (**a**) Asymmetrical channel set. (**b**) Asymmetrical channel index

## 4.8  Performance Evaluation

In this section, we evaluate the performance of the proposed algorithms in terms of reliability and broadcast delay. By reliability, we mean the percent of successful broadcast delivery within bounded time among multiple experiments. To that end, we choose the naive random broadcast algorithm, referred to as Random, as a benchmark where the sink and each node select their individual active slots based on their duty cycles and hop to a channel among their channel sets at random, because no existing work handles the multiple-channel broadcast problem in duty-cycling networks.

Specifically, we first illustrate the reliability of our broadcast algorithms and the random algorithm and then perform a series of simulations to evaluate the delay performance of three algorithms in several typical scenarios ranging from the synchronous single-channel case to the asynchronous and asymmetrical multi-channel case. In the simulation, node $a$ has the smallest duty cycle among all sensor nodes. Moreover, in multi-channel scenario, we may vary $N = 3, 5, 8$ corresponding to IEEE 802.15.6 [8] on low and high bands of UWB, respectively. Note that throughout the simulation, the broadcast delay is all calculated by the number of time slots.

### 4.8.1  Performance Comparison: Reliability

**MCB and Improved MCB Are Able to Guarantee the Success of Every Broadcast Task, While Random Fails Due to Its Probabilistic Nature**  Table 4.1 lists the reliability comparison of MCB, improved MCB, and Random in single-channel and multi-channel cases. All results are calculated from 4000 independent experiments under the simulation settings as in Sect. 4.8.2.

It is noticed that our MCB and improved MCB algorithms can achieve 100% reliability, meaning that they can ensure the successful broadcast delivery in single-channel and multi-channel cases within bounded broadcast delay. However, the reliability of Random is only 65.5% in single-channel case and it dramatically

**Table 4.1** Reliability of MCB, improved MCB, and random

| | Reliability | | | |
|---|---|---|---|---|
| | | Multi-channel | | |
| Algorithms | Single-channel | $N = 3$ | $N = 5$ | $N = 8$ |
| Random | 0.655 | 0.556 | 0.19 | 0.09 |
| MCB | 1 | 1 | 1 | 1 |
| Improved MCB | 1 | 1 | 1 | 1 |

decreases as the increase in the number of broadcast channels in multi-channel case. The main reason lies in that both MCB and improved MCB carefully tune the wake-up and channel hopping schedule to ensure that the sink and an arbitrary node overlap in at least one active slot.

Due to the unreliability of Random, for comparison, we calculate the broadcast delay of Random only in the cases where the successful broadcast delivery of Random happens among the 1000 experiments in the rest of this chapter.

### 4.8.2 Performance Comparison: Broadcast Delay

**Single-Channel Case** We now study the broadcast delay in single-channel case in terms of the worst-case and average broadcast delay which are the most and average broadcast delay among 1000 trials, respectively, under three representative scenarios depending on the duty cycles of $s$ and $a$:

- Both $s$ and $a$ have large duty cycles: $d_s = 10, d_a = 16$;
- Both of them have small duty cycles: $d_s = 50, d_a = 60$ and $d_s = 70, d_a = 90$;
- $s$ has large duty cycle, while $a$ has small duty cycle: $d_s = 10, d_a = 60$.

Note that the duty cycles of the other sensor nodes are not less than $\delta_a$.

Figures 4.4 and 4.5 show the worst-case broadcast delay and the average broadcast delay with any amount of clock drifts randomly distributed in $[1, T_s T_a]$ which is obtained by taking the average value of 1000 trials. From the simulation results, we can make the following observations:

- The broadcast delay increases as the reciprocal of duty cycles of $s$ or/and $a$, which is in accordance with the analytical results.
- In all simulation cases, the worst-case broadcast delay of MCB and improved MCB is bounded, which is in accordance with our theoretical result established in Theorem 4.3. However, as demonstrated in Table 4.1, Random cannot ensure the successful broadcast delivery within bounded delay, i.e., the worst-case broadcast delay of Random is not bounded.
- The improved MCB algorithm works better than the baseline MCB algorithm in terms of the worst-case broadcast delay and average broadcast delay. The main reason lies in that MCB uses only one pair of co-prime numbers to guarantee bounded broadcast delay even for asymmetrical duty cycles and the relative clock

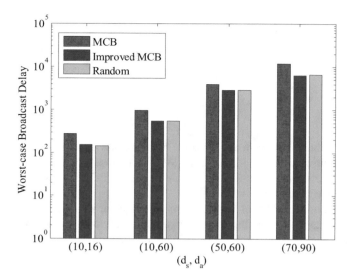

**Fig. 4.4** Single-channel: worst-case BD

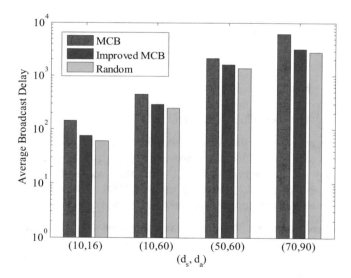

**Fig. 4.5** Single-channel: average BD

drifts. However, for the limited choices of co-prime numbers, the MCB restricts the duty cycle reciprocal of $s$ to a power-multiple of two, i.e., 2, 4, 8, etc. As a natural consequence, when the required duty cycle reciprocal deviates from the power-multiples, the related error increases significantly, leading to the larger broadcast delay of MCB. In contrast, the improved MCB exploits two pairs of co-prime numbers to improve the duty cycle granularity which has been proved in Lemma 4.1 and thus can significantly decrease the broadcast delay, especially in the unlucky case.

- The differences between the worst-case and average broadcast delay of MCB and improved MCB are slight under small duty cycles while becoming relatively obvious under large duty cycles, which is due to the pronounced negative impact of approximating the duty cycle reciprocal of 10 by a power-multiple 16 on the broadcast delay.

**Multi-Channel Case**  We move to performance evaluation in multi-channel scenario. Specifically, we trace the worst-case and average broadcast delay with full diversity by simulating the following two scenarios: $s$ and $a$ have the same or different channel perceptions.

**Both $s$ and $a$ Have the Same Channel Perception** i.e., $\mathcal{N}_s = \mathcal{N}_a = \mathcal{N}$. Figures 4.6 and 4.7 illustrate the worst-case and average broadcast delay with full diversity under asymmetric duty cycles and drifted slots when $N = 3$. The simulation results show similar characteristics as that in single-channel case: MCB and improved MCB achieve the bounded worst-case broadcast delay with full diversity but Random fails, which is in accordance with the result established in

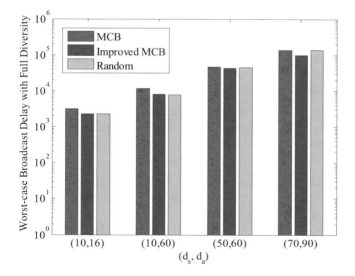

**Fig. 4.6**  Multi-channel: worst-case BD-FD

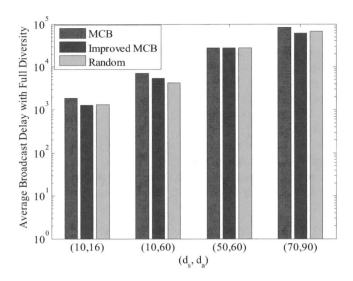

**Fig. 4.7** Multi-channel: average BD-FD

Table 4.1. Moreover, the broadcast delay with full diversity increases in proportion to the product of the reciprocals of the duty cycles of $s$ and $a$, which is in accordance with our theoretical results established in Theorem 4.4 with the constant number of broadcast channels. Another observation we can draw is that improved MCB performs best in guaranteeing the broadcast delivery with full diversity within less time under different duty cycles. More specifically, the performance difference in multi-channel becomes much more slight than that in single-channel case.

We proceed by evaluating the first successful broadcast delay which is the most time needed by the sink $s$ to successfully broadcast to for the first time all sensor nodes among the 1000 experiments in multi-channel case. From Figs. 4.8 and 4.9, we can also draw that the improved MCB algorithm globally performs best for all different duty cycles pairs.

Furthermore, we depict the worst-case and average broadcast delay with full diversity among all experiments with the fixed duty cycles (10,16) of $s$ and $a$ and the varying number of broadcast channels in Fig. 4.10. From the results, we make the following observations:

- As the system scales in terms of the channel set size $N$, the broadcast delay with full diversity also increases, specifically, at the square speed, which is in accordance with the analytical results.
- Improved MCB performs best in terms of both the worst-case and average broadcast delay while guaranteeing the successful broadcast delivery with full diversity within bounded broadcast delay. The results are in accordance with the theoretical analysis stated in Theorem 4.4. Although experiencing the lower

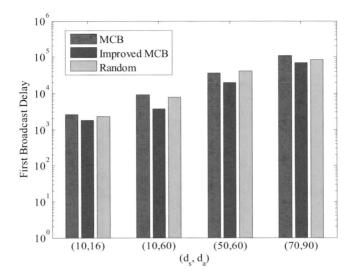

**Fig. 4.8** Multi-channel: worst-case first BD

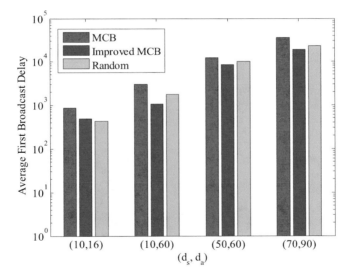

**Fig. 4.9** Multi-channel: average first BD

worst-case and average broadcast delay in some cases, Random cannot guarantee the successful deliveries in all experiments, which has been demonstrated by the reliability comparison in Table 4.1.

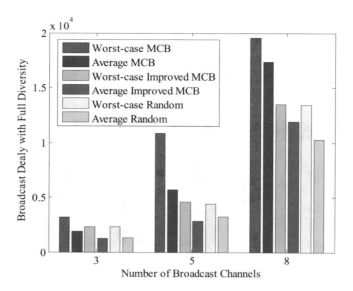

**Fig. 4.10** Broadcast delay with full diversity vs. the number of channels

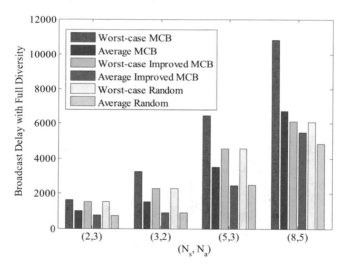

**Fig. 4.11** Asymmetrical channel perceptions: BD-FD

*s* **and** *a* **Have Asymmetrical Channel Perceptions** i.e., $\mathcal{N}_s \neq \mathcal{N}_a$. Figures 4.11 and 4.12 trace the worst-case and average broadcast delay with full diversity and for the first delivery with diverse channel perceptions, respectively. As shown in the pictures, improved MCB can achieve successful broadcast delivery on each common channel within less time though in the presence of asymmetrical channel

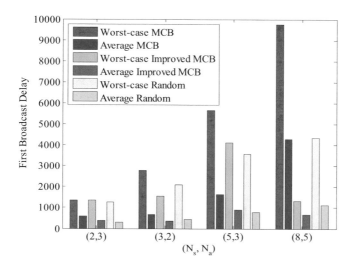

**Fig. 4.12** Asymmetrical channel perceptions: first BD

perceptions. This property of improved MCB makes it especially appropriate for the decentralized applications of WBSNs with heterogeneity between the sink and sensor nodes.

## 4.9  Conclusion

In this chapter, we have studied the multi-channel broadcast problem in duty-cycling WBSNs. The performance bound of any multi-broadcast algorithm has been derived. With the guidance of theoretical results, the MCB and improved MCB have been proposed to solve the problem, guaranteeing the successful broadcast delivery with full diversity regardless of the clock drifts and asymmetric duty cycles and channel perceptions within the order-minimal worst-case delay. Finally, the simulation results have demonstrated the superiority of the MCB and improved MCB in reliability and broadcast delay in several typical application scenarios.

## References

1. R. Zhang, H. Moungla, A. Mehaoua, An energy-efficient leader election mechanism for wireless body area networks, in *2014 IEEE Global Communications Conference* (IEEE, Piscataway, 2014), pp. 2411–2416
2. R. Zhang, H. Moungla, A. Mehaoua, A reliable and energy-efficient leader election algorithm for wireless body area networks, in *2015 IEEE International Conference on Communications (ICC)* (IEEE, Piscataway, 2015), pp. 530–535

3. D. Singelée, B. Latré, B. Braem, M. Peeters, M. De Soete, P. De Cleyn, B. Preneel, I. Moerman, C. Blondia, A secure low-delay protocol for wireless body area networks. Ad Hoc Sensor Wireless Netw. **9**(1–2), 53–72 (2010)
4. E. Rebeiz, G. Caire, A.F. Molisch, Energy-delay tradeoff and dynamic sleep switching for Bluetooth-like body-area sensor networks. IEEE Trans. Commun. **60**(9), 2733–2746 (2012)
5. R. Zhang, H. Moungla, A. Mehaoua, Delay analysis of IEEE 802.15. 6 CSMA/CA mechanism in duty-cycling WBANs, in *IEEE GLOBECOM 2015* (2015), pp. 1–6
6. R. Zhang, H. Moungla, J. Yu, et al., Medium access for concurrent traffic in wireless body area networks: protocol design and analysis. IEEE Trans. Veh. Technol., **66**(3), 2586–2599 (2016)
7. K. Han, J. Luo, Y. Liu, A.V. Vasilakos, Algorithm design for data communications in duty-cycled wireless sensor networks: a survey. IEEE Commun. Mag. **51**(7), 107–113 (2013)
8. I.S. Association et al., IEEE standard for local and metropolitan area networks-part 15.6: wireless body area networks. IEEE Stand. Inf. Technol. **802**(6), 1–271 (2012)
9. F. Wang, J. Liu, Duty-cycle-aware broadcast in wireless sensor networks, in *INFOCOM 2009, IEEE* (IEEE, Piscataway, 2009), pp. 468–476
10. X. Jiao, W. Lou, J. Ma, J. Cao, X. Wang, X. Zhou, Duty-cycle-aware minimum latency broadcast scheduling in multi-hop wireless networks, in *IEEE 30th International Conference on Distributed Computing Systems (ICDCS), 2010* (IEEE, Piscataway, 2010), pp. 754–763
11. X. Jiao, W. Lou, J. Ma, J. Cao, X. Wang, X. Zhou, Minimum latency broadcast scheduling in duty-cycled multihop wireless networks. IEEE Trans. Parallel Distrib. Syst. **23**(1), 110–117 (2012)
12. S. Guo, L. He, Y. Gu, B. Jiang, T. He, Opportunistic flooding in low-duty-cycle wireless sensor networks with unreliable links. IEEE Trans. Comput. **63**(11), 2787–2802 (2014)
13. L. Xu, G. Chen, J. Cao, S. Lin, H. Dai, X. Wu, F. Wu, Optimizing energy efficiency for minimum latency broadcast in low-duty-cycle sensor networks. ACM Trans. Sensor Netw. **11**(4), 57 (2015)
14. Y. Song, J. Xie, A distributed broadcast protocol in multi-hop cognitive radio ad hoc networks without a common control channel, in *Proceedings of IEEE INFOCOM, 2012* (IEEE, Piscataway, 2012), pp. 2273–2281
15. S. Dabideen, R. Ramanathan, W. Dron, A. Leung, Exploiting frequency groups for broadcasting in multi-channel multi-radio networks, in *2014 IEEE Military Communications Conference* (IEEE, Piscataway, 2014), pp. 1549–1555
16. J.-H. Lim, K. Naito, J.-H. Yun, M. Gerla, Revisiting overlapped channels: efficient broadcast in multi-channel wireless networks, in *2015 IEEE Conference on Computer Communications (INFOCOM)* (IEEE, Piscataway, 2015), pp. 1984–1992
17. L. Chen, K. Bian, X. Du, X. Li, Multichannel broadcast via channel hopping in cognitive radio networks. IEEE Trans. Veh. Technol. **64**(7), 3004–3017 (2015)
18. L. Chen, Z. Xiao, K. Bian, S. Shi, R. Li, Y. Ji, Skolem sequence based self-adaptive broadcast protocol in cognitive radio networks (2016). Preprint. arXiv:1602.00066
19. M.B. Nathanson, *Elementary Methods in Number Theory*, vol. 195 (Springer, Berlin, 2008)

# Chapter 5
# Energy-Efficient and Reliable Sleep Scheduling Algorithms in WBSNs

**Chapter Roadmap** The rest of this chapter is organized as follows: Section 5.1 explains the motivation of studying sleep scheduling problem and summarizes the contributions. Section 5.2 gives a brief overview of related work about sleep scheduling algorithms. Section 5.3 defines some preliminary knowledge. In Sect. 5.4, we describe the system model and formulates the maximum weighted $m$-fold dominating set problem. Then, we introduce two approximate algorithms and theoretically analyze their performance in Sects. 5.5 and 5.6. The performance of our proposed algorithms is evaluated in Sect. 5.7. Finally, we conclude the chapter in Sect. 5.8.

## 5.1 Introduction

### 5.1.1 Context and Motivation

Recent years have witnessed an unprecedented development of WBSNs that enable wireless and continuous medical monitoring of human body and significantly improve the healthcare efficiency. Typically, a WBSN comprises two types of devices: low-power sensor nodes and one sink. Sensor nodes are able to monitor real-time physiological parameters, such as heartbeat, temperature, electrocardiogram (ECG), and electroencephalogram (EEG) [1], while the sink collects data measured by the sensors and transmits them to specific users via wireless channels. Due to its promising applications in personalized medicine and home-based mobile health, WBSNs have drawn considerable research attention [2]. There are two main challenges, however, in deploying efficient and reliable WBSNs:

- *Limited energy resource*: Tiny sensors in WBSNs are generally equipped with very limited battery power. It is too difficult to recharge or replace the battery when its energy is depleted, especially for the one implanted in the body, energy

© Springer Nature Switzerland AG 2020

R. Zhang and J. Yu, *Energy-Efficient Algorithms and Protocols for Wireless Body Sensor Networks*, https://doi.org/10.1007/978-3-030-28580-7_5

efficiency should thus be the primary metric in WBSNs. In this context, one of the fundamental problems in WBSNs is how to prolong the network lifetime. The duty-cycling technique has been extensively regarded as an efficient solution to this problem [3]. In a duty-cycling WBSN, sensors can periodically alternate between active and sleep states. Although duty-cycling methods can remarkably save energy, they suffer severe delay as a sender has to wait for the wake-up of the receiver for data transmission. While in medical applications, data about physiological parameters should be transmitted in time such that physicians can make prompt diagnosis and treatment. Therefore, how to efficiently schedule sensor nodes to prolong the network lifetime while guaranteeing delay requirement is still an urgent challenge in WBSNs.

- *Unstable wireless channel*: Communication is unstable in WBSNs for two reasons. First, the path loss and shadowing effects for the prevalent absorption of human tissues may be very heavy in WBSNs [4]. Second, the human movement makes the wireless channel conditions among sensor nodes and between sensor nodes and the sink frequently changes with time [5]. Considering the heavy path loss, variable channel conditions in WBSNs, a pair of sensor nodes may fail to communicate even both in active states, which dramatically degrades the network performance. Thereby, it is desirable to maintain a certain degree of redundancy to enhance the network reliability, i.e., once waking up, each node needs to have more than one active neighbors that can receive their data.

Although considerable research efforts have been devoted to studying energy-efficient scheduling problem in WBSNs, the network reliability is overlooked. In this chapter, we aim to design efficient and reliable sleep scheduling algorithms for WBSNs. The key idea underlying our work is to selectively activate partial nodes in each given time frame, while the others can either wake up to transmit data or sleep to save energy according to their individual packet traffics. To address the limited energy resource and unstable wireless channel challenges, the sleep scheduling should follow the rules as below: The selected active nodes at each frame should form a dominating set (DS) such that each of the others connects with $m \geq 1$ selected nodes and can thus transmit data once it wakes up. Moreover, as the nodes in DS playing the role of relay nodes for the others need to keep active, they will suffer more load and energy consumption. Therefore, for each frame we construct a DS with minimum cardinality and maximum residual energy. As a result, the sleep scheduling in each frame can be formulated as a minimum weighted $m$-fold dominating set (MWmDS) problem that is proven NP-hard.

## 5.1.2   Summary of Contributions

To the best of our knowledge, our work is the first effort on sleep scheduling in WBSNs from the perspective of constructing MWmDS. The main contributions of this chapter are articulated as follows:

- First, we study the efficient and reliable sleep scheduling problem in WBSNs, and formulate it as the MWmDS problem and further show its NP-hardness.
- Second, we propose a global approximation algorithm (GAA) to construct an MWmDS by designing a polymatroid function and selecting the optimal node in the whole network each time. We analyze the performance of GAA and prove that its approximation ratio is $H(m + \delta)$, where $H(\cdot)$ is the harmonic number and $\delta$ is the maximum node degree.
- Third, we further design a local approximation algorithm (LAA) that selects one optimal node from each one-hop region each time and can add multiple nodes into the MWmDS at a time, reducing the computational complexity and recursive rounds of the algorithm compared to GAA. We prove that the upper bound of the approximation ratio of LAA is $1 + \ln(m\delta)$.
- Finally, the simulation results demonstrate the effectiveness and efficiency of our algorithms in terms of prolonging the network lifetime and constructing an MWmDS.

## 5.2   Related Work

In this section, we outline the existing work related to the sleep scheduling and summarize their limitations.

Duty cycling as an effective energy-saving technique is prevalently employed in WBSNs. A two-phase receiver-initiated duty-cycling protocol was presented in [6] for WBSNs which takes into consideration concurrent traffic to reduce the energy consumed by collisions, overhearing, and idle listening. In [7], the authors proposed a low duty-cycling protocol for WBSNs under low data-rate monitoring medical traffic to lower the energy consumed on beacon frames transmission. However, these protocols are mostly based on the fixed duty cycles. In practice, the traffic may be time varying in WBSNs depending on patients' conditions. Moreover, they fail to guarantee network reliability.

An energy-efficient scheduling problem was investigated in [8] through the Lyapunov optimization. The authors proposed a two-step scheduling algorithm where a sensor first decides whether or not to wake up based on the current queue state and network information statistics, then it estimates the channel condition and decides how much data to transmit after wakes up. As a result, the algorithm could guarantee a trade-off between the energy consumption and delay limit. Subsequently, the authors proposed a joint sleep scheduling and opportunistic transmission policy to minimize the average network energy consumption subject to the network stability in [9]. By tuning parameter in the Lyapunov optimization theory, this policy could reduce the average energy expenditure and stabilize the network queue length. However, these sleep scheduling methods work effectively only in one-hop WBSN, i.e., the sensor nodes transmit their data to the sink directly. While two-hop communication via a relay node is also specified in IEEE 802.15.6 standard [10], in order to overcome high path loss and enhance network reliability. As investigated in [11], it is effective of two-hop communication in improving network reliability in WBSNs.

For the two- or multiple-hop networks, scheduling sensor nodes is transferred to construct the connected dominating set (CDS) [12]. Since this problem is NP-hard, a significant amount of efforts are made to design a polynomial time heuristic or approximation algorithm. Specifically, the authors in [13] proposed a centralized algorithm and two distributed algorithms to construct a minimum size $km$-CDS. The simulation results showed that the proposed algorithms can construct a $km$-CDS with small size and with a high success rate. The authors in [14] and [15] introduced a new polynomial time factor approximation algorithm using the Tutte decomposition to construct a fault-tolerant CDS in unit disk graph. A constant approximation algorithm for the minimum weight $km$-CDS was presented in [16] under the assumption that $k$ and $m$ are two fixed constant with $m \geq k$. However, these algorithms are designed for unit disk graph where sensor nodes are assumed to have the same transmission range. If specific properties of unit disk graph cannot be satisfied, they cannot work. In practice, due to the independent energy constraint and individual applications of sensor nodes in WBSNs, the sensor nodes have heterogeneous transmission range. Although the authors presented a greedy algorithm in [17] to compute an $m$-fold CDS with performance ratio $2+\ln(\delta+m-2)$ in a general graph where $\delta$ is the maximum degree, they do not consider the impact of residual energy of sensors when constructing CDS. Moreover, they are not designed for WBSNs and ignore the nature of WBSNs, so they are inapplicable to WBSNs.

In summary, how to efficiently and reliably schedule sensor nodes to prolong the network lifetime in two-hop WBSNs is still an open challenge. Different from the existing work, we follow the guideline that the energy is the primary consideration in designing algorithms for WBSNs. To achieve energy-efficient and reliable sleep scheduling in a WBSN, we propose two algorithms that can find a DS with the minimum cardinality and maximum residual energy to optimize network lifetime.

## 5.3  Preliminary

In this section, we present preliminary knowledge on auxiliary definitions and results used in this chapter.

**Definition 5.1 ($m$-Fold Dominating Set)** A dominating set (DS) in a graph $G = (V, E)$ is a subset $D \subseteq V$ such that every node in $V - D$ is adjacent to at least one node in $D$. The nodes in DS are called **dominators**, while the non-DS nodes in the graph are call **dominatees**. A DS will be an **m-fold DS** if a subset $D \subseteq V$ such that every node in $V - D$ has at least $m$ neighbors in $D$.

**Definition 5.2 (Polymatroid Function)**  Consider a finite set $U$ and a function $f : 2^U \mapsto \mathbb{R}^+$, for any two sets $A$ and $B$ in $U$, the function is to be submodular if

$$f(A) + f(B) \geq f(A \cap B) + f(A \cup B).$$

Assume that $f$ is a submodular function on set $U$, for any two subsets $C, D \subseteq U$, let

$$\triangle_D f(C) = f(C \cup D) - f(C)$$

be a marginal profit obtained by adding subset $D$ to $C$. For simplicity, when $D = \{x\}$ is a single node, $\triangle_x f(C)$ will be used to denote $\triangle_{\{x\}} f(C)$. Then, the function $f$ is submodular and monotone increasing if and only if, for any two subsets $C \subseteq D \subseteq U$ and any $x \in (U - D)$,

$$\triangle_x f(C) \geq \triangle_x f(D)$$

holds. A monotone increasing and submodular function $f$ with $f(\varnothing) = 0$ is called a **polymatroid function**.

**Definition 5.3 (Minimum Submodular Cover Problem)**  Consider a submodular function $f$, let $\Omega_f = \{C \subseteq U \mid \triangle_x f(C) = 0, \text{ for any } x \in (U - C)\}$. $\Omega_f$ contains the maximal set $C$ under function $f$, in other words, the marginal profit cannot increase by adding any node $x$ into subset $C$. Given a finite set $U$, a polymatroid function $f$, and a nonnegative cost function $c$ on $U$, the minimum submodular cover problem can be formulated as follows:

$$\text{minimize} \quad c(C) = \sum_{x \in C} c(x)$$

$$\text{subject to} \quad C \in \Omega_f.$$

To address the minimum submodular cover problem, given a polymatroid function $f$, one can design a greedy algorithm with the performance as stated in the following lemma [18].

**Lemma 5.1**  *The greedy algorithm using a polymatroid function $f$ for the submodular cover problem produces an approximation solution with approximation ratio $H(\gamma)$, where $\gamma = \max\limits_{x \in U} f(\{x\})$ and $H(\gamma) = \sum_{i=1}^{\gamma} \frac{1}{i}$ is the harmonic number.*

## 5.4   System Model and Problem Statement

### 5.4.1   System Model

In a WBSN, the sensor nodes are usually deployed in the appropriate places based on their individual functionalities, and the only one sink is generally located on the belly of human body, as shown in Fig. 5.1. Let $G = (V, E)$ denote a WBSN, where $V = \{1, 2, \cdots, N\}$ is the set of sensor nodes, $N$ denotes the network size, and $E$ is the set of edges denoting the neighborhood relationship among all sensor nodes. In the WBSN, we assume that the sink is always active and is supposed to have adequate energy, and a sensor node can communicate with the sink in two hops via a relay node, as specified in IEEE 802.15.6 standard [10]. For each sensor node $v \in V$, $\mathbb{N}(v)$ denotes the set of the neighbor nodes of $v$ in $V$, and $w_v(t)$ defines its residual energy at time $t$. Note that $w_v(0)$ is the initial energy of node $v$, and the energy consumption mode [19] for $v$ to transmit and receive $l$-bits data over distance $d$ along the surface of the human body is exploited as follows:

$$\begin{cases} E_{Tx}(l, d, n) & = l E_{Txelec} + l \epsilon_{amp}(n) d^n \\ E_{Rx}(l) & = l E_{Rxelec} \end{cases}, \tag{5.1}$$

where $E_{Txelec}$ and $E_{Rxelec}$ are the energy dissipated to run the circuitry by radio in order to transmit and receive, respectively, and $\epsilon_{amp}$ is the energy consumption to amplify the transmission. $d$ is the distance between the transmitter and the receiver, and $n$ denotes the path loss coefficient. The *lifetime* of a sensor node is defined as duration from when it starts working to when its energy is depleted. In other words, if $t$ is the first time when $w_v(t) \leq 0$, $v$ cannot work anymore and its lifetime is $t$.

Without loss of generality, the work period of a WBSN is divided into a series of time frames. At the beginning of each frame, we select partial sensor nodes to form a DS and have them stay active in this frame, while the unselected nodes will turn off their radio to save energy. For example, in a given frame, the sensor nodes $\{3, 5, 8, 14, 15\}$ are chosen to work, while other sensor nodes $\{1, 2, 4, 6, 7, 9, 10, 11, 12, 13, 16\}$ can go to sleep based on the topology in Fig. 5.1. Note that these sleeping nodes can still promptly switch to active state to monitor and transmit data upon their individual traffics. As the nodes in DS suffer from more energy consumption, which will lead to rapid death, it is necessary to switch to a fresh DS from frame to frame to prolong the network lifetime. For example, we can build a new DS of sensor nodes $\{2, 6, 7, 10, 16\}$ to replace the previous one to work in a new frame. Thereby, we formally define the *network lifetime* of a WBSN as follows:

**Definition 5.4 (Network Lifetime)** Let $T_s$ be the frame that the network $G$ starts to work, and $T_d$ be the frame when there does not exist any DS in G. Then, the network lifetime can be expressed by $T = T_d - T_s$.

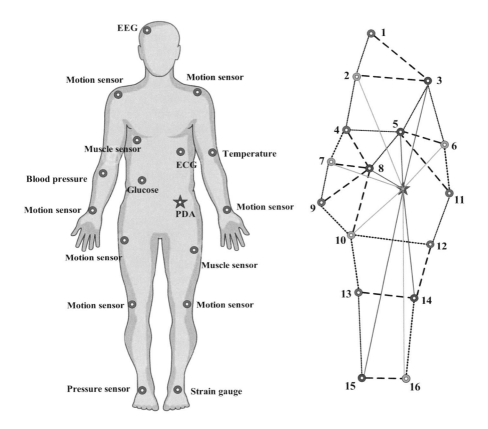

**Fig. 5.1**  The sensor deployment in a WBSN

## 5.4.2   Problem Formulation

The sleep scheduling scheme in this chapter is to construct a DS for each frame such that the network lifetime is maximized. Consider the following characteristics of WBSNs: (1) *More energy burden on dominator nodes*: as the nodes in DS that play the role of relay nodes have to keep active and may aggregate data packets from dominatees, they will have extra energy consumption. (2) *Unstable wireless channel*: due to severe path loss and time-varying channel conditions in WBSNs resulted from high absorption of human tissues and human movement, a pair of neighbors may fail to communicate even both in active state, which will degrade the network performance. Therefore, we should construct such a DS that has two properties: On the one hand, it comprises the minimum number of nodes and has maximum residual energy, seeking lifetime maximization; on the other hand, the DS is $m$-fold to ensure high reliability, that is to say, each node needs to have $m$ active neighbors, i.e., relay nodes, and can choose the optimal one to send data. In nature, the key of efficient and reliable sleep scheduling is to construct a minimum weighted $m$-fold dominating set (MWmDS) for each frame.

Given a WBSN $G$ and the residual energy of each node $w_v(t)$, we aim to construct an $m$-fold DS, denoted by $S$, which satisfies the requirement of $\Omega_f$ in $V$ and has the maximum residual energy. Mathematically, from Definition 5.3, the MWmDS problem can be expressed as

$$\text{minimize} \quad W(S) = \sum_{v \in S} \frac{1}{w_v(t)}$$

$$\text{subject to} \quad S \in \Omega_f. \tag{5.2}$$

Given such a DS $S$, the nodes in $S$ will keep active, while the other nodes in $V - S$ which have $m$ neighbors in $S$ can either be active or sleep depending on their individual traffics.

The challenge here lies in the combinatorial nature of the MWmDS problem. When dissecting this problem, we find it NP-hard and formally state the observation below.

**Theorem 5.1** *The MWmDS problem is NP-hard.*

*Proof* Let $m = 1$, then the MWmDS problem can be transformed to the minimum weighted dominating set problem which has been proven to be NP-hard in [20]. Therefore, the MWmDS problem is also NP-hard.                    □

Due to the NP-hardness of the MWmDS problem, we need to design algorithms, trying to approach the optimal solution. With the guidance of polymatroid function in Definition 5.2, in what follows, we will first present an approximation algorithm, namely GAA, to find MWmDS. We then develop a simplified algorithm, referred to as LAA, which significantly reduces the computational complexity of GAA.

## 5.5  GAA: Global Approximation Algorithm

In this section, we elaborate an approximation algorithm that can construct an MWmDS for a WBSN, and then analyze the algorithm performance.

---

**Algorithm 1** GAA: constructing MWmDS

---

**Input**: $G(V, E), m$
**Output**: MWmDS

1: $S \leftarrow \varnothing, q_1 = 0, q_2 = 0$
2: **repeat**
3: **for** each $v \in (V - S)$ **do**
4:     computes its neighbors $N_S(v)$ in $S$
5:     **if** $|N_S(v)| < m$ **then**
6:         $q_1 = q_1 + (m - |N_S(v)|)$
7:     **end if**
8: **end for**
9: **for** each $v \in (V - S)$ **do**
10:     **for** each $u \in (V - (S \cup v))$ **do**
11:         computes its neighbors $N_{(S \cup v)}(u)$ in $(S \cup v)$
12:         **if** $|N_{(S \cup v)}(u)| < m$ **then**
13:             $q_2 = q_2 + (m - |N_{(S \cup v)}(u)|)$
14:         **end if**
15:     **end for**
16: **end for**
17: **for** each $v \in (V - S)$ **do**
18:     select the node $v$ with maximum $(q_1 - q_2)^\alpha \cdot w_v(t)^{(1-\alpha)}$
19: **end for**
20: $S \leftarrow (S \cup v)$
21: **until** there does not exist a node $v \in (V - S)$ such that $\triangle_v Q(S) > 0$

---

## 5.5.1 Algorithm Design

For a node $v \in (V - S)$, let $\mathbb{N}_S(v)$ denote the set of neighbors of node $v$ in set $S$, and $|\mathbb{N}_S(v)|$ define its cardinality. Suppose that each node in $V - S$ has at least $m$ neighbors to be active in $S$, where $m \geq 1$. Denote by $g_S(v)$ the times that node $v$ needs to be dominated, we can calculate $g_S(v)$ as

$$g_S(v) = \begin{cases} \max\{m - |\mathbb{N}_S(v)|, 0\} & v \in V - S \\ 0 & v \in S \end{cases}. \qquad (5.3)$$

Note that, in order to satisfy the constraints in MWmDS problem, the $|\mathbb{N}_S(v)|$ of an arbitrary node $v \in (V - S)$ should be at least equal to $m$ at the end of the algorithm execution. Given the required number $m$, the total remaining domination requirement of the whole network can thus be calculated by

$$Q(S) = mN - \sum_{v \in S} g_S(v). \qquad (5.4)$$

Recall the definition of polymatroid function, if one node $v$ is added to the solution set $S$, which brings a positive marginal profit of degree, i.e., $\triangle_v Q(S) > 0$, the node should be selected as a potential dominator. Since the lifetime of a WBSN depends on the residual energy of sensor nodes, we should take into consideration the residual energy when building an MWmDS. Consequently, we require that only the optimal potential dominator $v$ that can maximize $\triangle_v Q(S)^\alpha \cdot w_v(t)^{(1-\alpha)}$ will finally become a dominator and is added to set $S$ in each iteration. Note that $\alpha \in (0, 1]$ is the weight factor that indicates the preference for the marginal profit of degree or the residual energy. In particular, $\alpha = 1$ implies the marginal profit of degree is the only criterion to be the dominator. As the marginal profit of degree indicates the network reliability, the value of $\alpha$ should be greater than 0 in order to guarantee the reliability. We will evaluate the impact of $\alpha$ on the network lifetime in the simulation.

In essence, the main idea of GAA is to globally select the node with optimal profit of node degree and residual energy to the dominator set in each iteration. More specifically, the nodes with positive marginal profit of degree are firstly added to a potential dominator set as lines 3–16 in Algorithm 1. Then, the optimal node $v$ which maximizes the product of marginal profit of degree $\triangle_v Q(S)^\alpha$ and residual energy $w_v(t)^{(1-\alpha)}$ is added to the final solution set $S$ in lines 17–20. The algorithm will not terminate until the marginal profit of degree does not increase, i.e., no new node can be added to $S$, thus the set $S$ satisfies the requirement of $\Omega_f$ and is an approximation to the MWmDS. The elaborated executable algorithm description is shown in Algorithm 1.

### 5.5.2  Algorithm Analysis

We analyze the algorithm performance and state the main properties and results in the following lemmas and theorems.

**Lemma 5.2** *Function $Q(S)$ is a polymatroid function.*

*Proof* From Eq. (5.4), it is easy to observe the fact that $Q(\varnothing)$ will be equal to 0, if $S = \varnothing$. On the other hand, we can also find from Eq. (5.3) that for any $v \in V$, function $-g_S(v)$ is monotone increasing with respect to $S$. Moreover, for any two subsets $C \subseteq D \subseteq V$ and for any node $u \in (V - D)$, we have $-\triangle_u g_C(v) \geq -\triangle_u g_D(v)$, implying that function $-g_S(v)$ is monotone increasing and is a submodular function. Consequently, function $Q(S)$ that is the sum of a constant function and monotone increasing and submodular functions is also monotone increasing and submodular. From the analysis above, function $Q(S)$ satisfies all properties listed in Definition 5.2, it is thus a polymatroid function.    □

**Lemma 5.3** *The constructed set $S$ in Algorithm 1 is an m-fold dominating set of graph $G$.*

*Proof* We prove this lemma via contradiction. First, suppose the existence of a node $u \in (V - S)$ with $|\mathbb{N}_S(u)| \leq m$, we have $\triangle_u g_S(u) = g_{S \cup u}(u) - g_S(u) = 0 - (m - |\mathbb{N}_S(u)|) < 0$. As $-g_S(v)$ is monotone increasing with respect to $S$, it holds that

$- \triangle_u g_S(v) \geq 0$ for any $v \in (V - u)$ and thus $\triangle_u Q(S) = - \sum_{v \in V} \triangle_u g_S(v) > 0$, implying that the algorithm would continue running in this case.                    □

**Theorem 5.2**  *The approximation ratio of Algorithm 1 is $H(m + \delta)$ to the optimal value opt for the MWmDS problem, where $\delta$ is the maximum degree of graph G.*

*Proof*  Since the MWmDS problem can be regarded as a special submodular cover problem as showed in Lemmas 5.2 and 5.3, we can address this problem by designing a greedy algorithm and a polymatroid function according to Lemma 5.1. It has been proven in Lemma 5.2 that the designed function $Q(S)$ satisfies the properties of the polymatroid function, thus we know that the weight of our solution is not bigger than $H(\gamma) \cdot opt$, where *opt* is the optimal value for the MWmDS problem and $\gamma = \max_{v \in V}\{Q(v)\} = \max_{v \in V}\{m|V| - \sum_{u \in (V-v)}(m - |\mathbb{N}_v(u)|)\} = \max_{v \in V}\{m + d_G(v)\} = m + \delta$, where $d_G(v)$ is the degree for any node $v$ in $G$. Note that $H(m + \delta) \leq 1 + \ln(m + \delta)$.                    □

**Theorem 5.3**  *The computational complexity of Algorithm 1 is $O(N^3)$, where N is the network size.*

*Proof*  As stated in Algorithm 1, we should first compute the total remaining domination requirement $Q(S)$ of the network with complexity $O(N)$ at each iteration. Then, in order to pick the optimal node and add it to the set $S$, we need to calculate the marginal profit $\triangle_v Q(S)$ of each unselected nodes in $O(N^2)$ steps. Subsequently, the node with maximum $\triangle_v Q(S)^\alpha \cdot w_v(t)^{(1-\alpha)}$ is picked with complexity $O(N)$. At last, the iteration will end when there does not exist any node that can bring the positive marginal profit. Therefore, the computational complexity of Algorithm 1 is $O(N)[O(N) + O(N^2) + O(N)] = O(N^3)$.                    □

## 5.6   LAA: Local Approximation Algorithm

With Algorithm 1, we can find an MWmDS that exceeds the optimal one as many as $H(m + \delta)$ with the computational complexity $O(N^3)$. In this section, we intend to present another algorithm that is able to achieve good performance with lower computational complexity.

### 5.6.1   Algorithm Design

Through analyzing Algorithm 1, we observe its two disadvantages. First, only one node can be selected as a dominator and be added to DS in each iteration, which is inefficient as the network scales. Second, the dominatees have to keep computing their marginal profit of degree to compete as dominators repeatedly even they already have at least $m$ neighbors in the found DS, which leads to high computational complexity and excessive execution rounds. To overcome these deficiencies, we introduce LAA that outputs multiple dominators in one iteration and reduces the number of the sensor nodes to be chosen significantly round after round.

LAA selects one dominator in each one-hop region via a coloring process. Assume that initially the colors of all nodes are white. If a node is selected as a dominator, it will be colored black. Correspondingly, once a node becomes a dominatee, its color will change from white to grey. Before the formal algorithm description, we first introduce a criterion, referred to as *domination capability* that is defined as follows.

**Definition 5.5 (Domination Capability)** The domination capability $D^c$ of a node is defined as the number of its white neighbors. The $D^c$ of $v$ is denoted by $D_v^c = |\{u|(u \in \mathbb{N}(v)) \cap color_u = white\}|$.

We next describe the proposed LAA that is formally stated in Algorithm 2. Initially, all nodes are white. Using these nodes as input, the algorithm will produce a DS consisting of all dominators that are colored black. In each round of the algorithm, the nodes with the highest domination capability and the most residual energy among one-hop neighbors will be selected as dominators and be added to DS. If there are more than one nodes with the same domination capability, the node with the most residual energy among them will be preferentially selected as a dominator. More specifically, as shown in Algorithm 2, if node $v$ has a strict higher domination capability and residual energy than all its white neighbors $u$, it will be a dominator. If there exists white neighbor $u$ that has the same domination capability as that of node $v$, $v$ has more residual energy than that of $u$, then, node $v$ can also be added to DS. In case that their residual energy are also the same, the node with the smaller ID between them will be singled out. In the case that node $v$ has lower domination capability and higher residual energy, it cannot become a dominator unless it has the maximum $(D_v^c)^\beta \cdot w_v(t)^{(1-\beta)}$, where $\beta \in (0, 1]$ expresses the favorable weight for the domination capability or the residual energy. Particularly, when $\beta = 1$, it indicates the totally preference for the domination capability, and the impact of $\beta$ on network lifetime will be assessed in the following simulation. Once none of $v$'s neighbors is white, i.e., the domination capability of node $v$ is zero, node $v$ has to be a dominator and added to DS. All the four conditions under one of which one node can become a dominator are described in step 5 of Algorithm 2. After that, all the selected dominators in the current round will change their color from white to black. Then, the remaining white nodes judge whether they have at least $m$ neighbors in current DS or not. If so, they will become dominatees and their colors become grey. Otherwise their colors stay white.

One thing worth noting is that there would be multiple nodes becoming dominators or dominatees in each round of LAA algorithm. Subsequently, the chosen dominators and dominatees in the current round are pruned, as a consequence, the number of white nodes input to the next round will remarkably decrease, which dramatically reduces the computational complexity in the next iteration. This algorithm will terminate at the moment that all nodes become black or grey, i.e., they are either dominators or dominatees.

## 5.6.2   Algorithm Analysis

In this subsection, we start analyzing the correctness and the efficiency of Algorithm 2.

**Lemma 5.4**  *All black nodes resulting from Algorithm 2 form an m-fold dominating set of graph G.*

*Proof*  It is easy to check that the set constructed by the black nodes is an $m$-fold DS, since the nodes in the network are all black or grey, and every grey node connects with at least $m$ black nodes after the execution of Algorithm 2. Suppose that there still exists a white node when Algorithm 2 ends. According to the execution

---

**Algorithm 2** LAA: constructing MWmDS

---

**Input**: $G(V, E)$ consisting of white nodes, $m$
**Output**: MWmDS consisting of black nodes
 1:  $S \leftarrow \varnothing, SE \leftarrow \varnothing, k \leftarrow 1$
 2:  **while** there exists a white node in $V$ **do**
 3:  $\quad R_k \leftarrow \varnothing, RE_k \leftarrow \varnothing$
 4:  $\quad$ **for** All white nodes $v \in V$ **do**
 5:  $\quad\quad$ **if** $v$ satisfies any one of the following conditions:
 $\quad\quad\quad$ (i) $D_v^c \geq D_u^c$ and $w_v(t) > w_u(t)$, where $u \in \mathbb{N}(v)$ and $color_u$=white
 $\quad\quad\quad$ (ii) $D_v^c = D_u^c$ and $w_v(t) = w_u(t)$ and $ID_v < ID_u$
 $\quad\quad\quad$ (iii) $(D_v^c)^\beta \cdot w_v(t)^{(1-\beta)} > (D_u^c)^\beta \cdot w_u(t)^{(1-\beta)}$
 $\quad\quad\quad$ (iv) $D_v^c = 0$
 $\quad\quad\quad$ **then**
 6:  $\quad\quad\quad$ Add $v$ to $R_k$
 7:  $\quad\quad\quad$ Change state of $v$ as dominator
 8:  $\quad\quad\quad$ Change color of $v$ from white to black
 9:  $\quad\quad$ **end if**
10:  $\quad$ **end for**
11:  $\quad S \leftarrow S \cup R_k$
12:  $\quad$ **for** All white nodes $u \in (V - S)$ **do**
13:  $\quad\quad$ Compute the neighbors $\mathbb{N}_s(u)$ in $S$
14:  $\quad\quad$ **if** $|\mathbb{N}_s(u)| \geq m$ **then**
15:  $\quad\quad\quad$ Add $u$ to $RE_k$
16:  $\quad\quad\quad$ Change state of $u$ as dominatee
17:  $\quad\quad\quad$ Change color of $u$ from white to grey
18:  $\quad\quad$ **end if**
19:  $\quad$ **end for**
20:  $\quad SE \leftarrow SE \cup RE_k$
21:  $\quad k \leftarrow k + 1$
22: **end while**

---

condition of the while loop in step 2 of Algorithm 2, the algorithm will not terminate in the presence of a white node. The white node will thus change to black or grey at last. This means that the assumption we made above does not hold. Therefore, the black nodes in $S$ form an $m$-fold DS. $\qquad\square$

**Theorem 5.4** *The upper bound of approximation ratio of Algorithm 2 is* $1+\ln(m\delta)$, *where* $\delta$ *is the maximum degree of graph G.*

*Proof* Let $opt$ be an optimal DS in $G$. At first, we construct a new graph $G'$ by duplicating each node of the original graph $G$ $m$ times. As a result, $G'$ has $mN$ nodes and its maximum node degree is $m\delta$. Then, we iteratively choose the optimal node into the set $S$. Note that the initial state of $S$ is $S = \phi$. The iteration will continue until the number of the remaining white nodes is less than the number of nodes in $opt$. And these remaining nodes will be eventually added to $S$. In the worst case, there is only one node to become a dominator in each iteration. Suppose that there are still $U_i$ white nodes after $i$-th iteration, we have

$$U_{i-1} - U_i \geq \frac{U_{i-1}}{opt}, \qquad i = 1, 2, 3, \ldots, \qquad (5.5)$$

where $U_0 = mN$. Following Eq. (5.5), we can derive that

$$U_i \leq U_{i-1}\left(1 - \frac{1}{opt}\right) \leq \cdots \leq U_0\left(1 - \frac{1}{opt}\right)^i.$$

As the iteration will stop when $U_i \geq opt$ while $U_{i+1} < opt$, we have

$$U_0\left(1 - \frac{1}{opt}\right)^i \geq U_i \geq opt.$$

Thus, according to the Taylor series for $e^{-\frac{1}{opt}}$, it holds that

$$i \leq opt \cdot \log(m\delta).$$

Then, we can have that the number of node in DS is

$$|S| \leq opt\,(1 + \ln(m\delta)).$$

Since the result above is derived in the worst case, the upper bound of approximation ratio of Algorithm 2 is $1 + \ln(m\delta)$. $\qquad\square$

**Theorem 5.5** *The computational complexity of Algorithm 2 is* $O(N^2)$.

*Proof* In Algorithm 2, each node first compares with its one-hop neighbors in terms of domination capability or residual energy within $O(N)$ operations in each round in order to become a dominator. Then, for the remaining white nodes, at most $O(N)$

operations are conducted to get the number of their individual neighbors in DS. The while loop will end once there is no white node. Therefore, the computational complexity of Algorithm 2 is equal to $O(N)[O(N) + O(N)] = O(N^2)$.                    □

## 5.7 Performance Evaluation

In this section, we use Matlab simulator to conduct performance evaluation. Since this chapter is the first effort on efficient and reliable sleep scheduling via constructing MWmDS in WBSNs, in order to show the effectiveness and efficiency of the sleep scheduling, we compare with the communication strategy without sensor sleep scheduling, referred to as Baseline, in the simulation.

### 5.7.1  Simulation Settings and Performance Metrics

Following the specification of IEEE 802.15.16 standard that one WBSN can support up to 256 sensors for biomedical applications [10], we vary the number of nodes in a WBSN from 10 to 120 in the simulation. We list the other simulation parameters in Table 5.1. More specifically, $E_{DA}$ defines the extra energy consumption of the dominators to aggregate data packets from dominatees. In the simulation, every result is given by the average of 100 independent experiments.

To comprehensively evaluate the performance, we assess the proposed algorithms with the following metrics:

- *Network lifetime*: In the beginning of each frame, a DS will be built to work and the nodes not in the DS can switch to sleep mode to conserve energy. Based on Definition 5.4, the network lifetime is defined as the frame until there does not exist any DS in the network. To justify the improvement of our sleep scheduling algorithms, the network lifetime is investigated in two scenarios.
- *Cardinality of DS*: The DS size, indicating the approximation ratio of GAA and LAA algorithms, is evaluated to verify the theoretical results in Theorems 5.2 and 5.4.

**Table 5.1** Simulation settings

| Parameter | Setting |
|---|---|
| Initial energy | 0.1 J |
| $E_{Txelec}$, $E_{Rxelec}$ | 16.7 nJ/bit, 36.1 nJ/bit |
| $\epsilon_{amp}(n)$ | 1.97 nJ/(bit m$^n$), ($n = 3.11$) |
| $E_{DA}$ | 5 nJ/bit/signal |
| Data packet size | 4000 bits |

- *Execution rounds*: Since the capability of sensor nodes in WBSNs is limited, the execution time in rounds spent constructing a DS is investigated to justify the efficiency of GAA and LAA algorithms.

### 5.7.2   Simulation Results

*(1) The impact of $\alpha$ and $\beta$*  In our MWmDS construction algorithms, the value of $\alpha$ and $\beta$ indicates the preference of the algorithm for the node degree or residual energy of each node during the final dominator election. Thus, we need to adopt an optimal value of $\alpha$ and $\beta$ for the network lifetime maximization.

In the first group of simulations, we evaluate the impact of $\alpha$ in GAA algorithm on the network lifetime. All nodes have 0.1 J of initial energy, and the energy consumption model in Eq. (5.1) is employed. Let $m = 1$, we consider three scenarios according to the network size that varies from 20 to 60 with an increasing step of 20. In each scenario, there are three kinds of networks with the same size but different average degrees of nodes: (a) smaller than half of the number of nodes, (b) equal to half of the number of nodes, (c) greater than half of the number of nodes. Figure 5.2 shows the results of the network lifetime under different values of $\alpha$ in three scenarios, respectively. Note that, in order to ensure the network reliability, the results plotted in Fig. 5.2 when $\alpha = 0$ are actually the values when $\alpha = 0.005$.

As shown in these figures, we can see that the network lifetime is maximum when $\alpha \in [0.1, 0.2]$. The maximum network lifetime exceeds the one when $\alpha = 1$ (i.e., the marginal profit of degree is the only criterion to choose the final dominator) by 38%, 15% and 8% on average in the three scenarios, respectively. The results demonstrate that the residual energy plays an important role in constructing MWmDS in GAA algorithm, and it is more important than marginal profit of degree

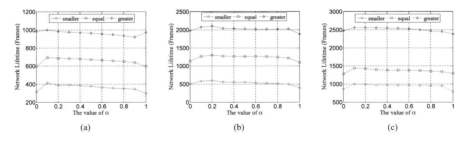

(a)                              (b)                              (c)

**Fig. 5.2**  The impact of $\alpha$ on the network lifetime under different network sizes: (**a**) 20 nodes, (**b**) 40 nodes, (**c**) 60 nodes ("smaller" in the legend means the average node degree is smaller than half of the number of nodes; "equal" means the former is equal to the latter; "greater" means the former is greater than the latter)

**Fig. 5.3** The impact of $\beta$ on the network lifetime under the network with 40 nodes ("smaller" in the legend means the average node degree is smaller than half of the number of nodes; "equal" means the former is equal to the latter; "greater" means the former is greater than the latter)

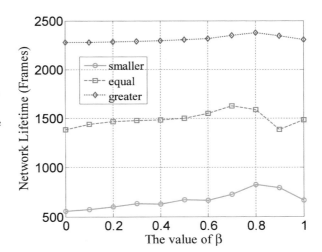

in terms of prolonging the network lifetime. Based on the observations, for the GAA algorithm, we set $\alpha = 0.15$ in the following simulations.

Then, we assess the impact of $\beta$ on the network lifetime for LAA algorithm. Similarly, the network lifetime with different values of $\beta$ is depicted in Fig. 5.3 when the network size is 40 nodes. We can find that the network lifetime achieves the maximum value as $\beta \in [0.7, 0.8]$, and it is 47%, 17%, and 5% larger than the minimum value when $\beta = 0.005$ (i.e., the residual energy is the only criterion to elect the dominator). Thus, it is proper to set the value of $\beta$ to be within [0.7, 0.8] for LAA algorithm, which demonstrates that the domination capability plays a more important role than residual energy in order to maximize the network lifetime. The main reason is that the domination capability that denotes the number of unscheduled nodes is updated with the execution of LAA algorithm in new topology after pruning the elected dominators and dominatees. The marginal profit of degree in GAA algorithm, however, is determined by the degree of each node which is fixed in original network. Therefore, the residual energy is more precedence in GAA algorithm, while LAA algorithm favors the domination capability. In the following simulations, we set $\beta = 0.75$.

*(2) The Network Lifetime* In the second part of simulation, we compare GAA and LAA algorithms with Baseline to show the superiority of sleep scheduling in terms of network lifetime. The network size varies from 10 to 100, and two types of node energy distribution are considered: (a) uniform distribution where each node has 0.1 J initial energy, (b) random distribution where each node is assigned a random initial energy from [0.1, 0.5].

Figures 5.4 and 5.5 illustrate that our MWmDS construction-based sleep scheduling GAA and LAA algorithms perform better than Baseline in prolonging the network lifetime even with $m = 2$ or 3 when the network can tolerate failure once or twice for each dominatee. Moreover, as $m = 2$ (or 3), the network lifetime

achieved by GAA algorithm is 306% (or 107%) longer than that achieved by
Baseline on average in Fig. 5.4 with uniform energy distribution. Correspondingly,
LAA algorithm is 232% (or 79%) better than Baseline as setting $m = 2$ (or 3). The
similar conclusions can be obtained from Fig. 5.5. These observations demonstrate
that our proposed sleep scheduling schemes are highly energy-efficient and reliable.
Furthermore, we can also find that the network lifetime of GAA is longer than that of
LAA although GAA takes more execution rounds to build a DS as shown in Fig. 5.7.
The main reason is that GAA can construct a globally optimal MWmDS based on
the whole network information for each frame, thus the cardinality of DS of GAA is
much smaller than that of LAA as shown in Fig. 5.6. However, LAA construct DS
is only based on one-hop neighbors information, so it is locally optimal. Thereby,

**Fig. 5.4** The network
lifetime with uniform energy
distribution

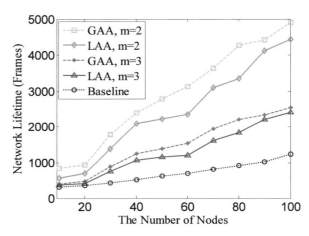

**Fig. 5.5** The network
lifetime with random energy
distribution

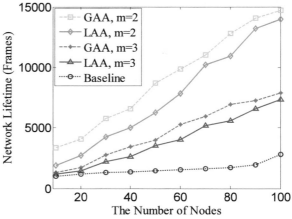

**Fig. 5.6** The cardinality of DS

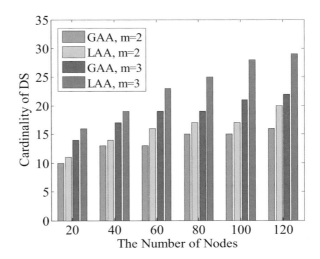

**Fig. 5.7** The execution rounds to build a DS

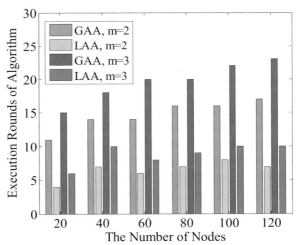

LAA may consume much more energy than that of GAA in each frame as a result of larger cardinality of DS.

*(3) Cardinality and Execution Rounds of DS* We then investigate the fundamental properties of GAA and LAA algorithms. To this end, we record the cardinality and the execution rounds taken to construct an MWmDS with $m = 2$ and $m = 3$. From the results shown in Figs. 5.6 and 5.7, respectively, we make the following observations:

- First, the constructed MWmDS scales with the increase of the network size and the value of $m$. With fixed $m$, GAA builds a smaller DS than LAA, which is in accordance with the analytical results in Theorems 5.2 and 5.4. The main reason is that the globally optimal node is selected each time in GAA, while LAA picks the locally optimal node in each one-hop region. For example, when $m = 3$, an MWmDS constructed by GAA consists of 22 nodes, while the number is extended to 29 for LAA in a network with 120 nodes.

- Second, LAA spends less time constructing an MWmDS than GAA as depicted in Fig. 5.7. This can be interpreted as follows. In LAA, multiple nodes from one-hop regions can be selected into MWmDS in each iteration instead of only one node in GAA such that LAA has fewer nodes input to the next iteration than GAA. For example, setting $m = 3$ for a network with 120 nodes, LAA runs only 10 rounds to construct an MWmDS, while GAA needs 22 rounds, more than two times the rounds of LAA.

## 5.8   Conclusion

In this chapter, we have studied the energy-efficient and reliable sleep scheduling problem in WBSNs via constructing minimum weighted $m$-fold dominating set (MWmDS). We first showed the NP-hardness of MWmDS construction problem and introduced an approximation algorithm, called GAA, which globally selected an optimal node that contributes to the maximum increment of a polymatroid function and residual energy to be the final dominator in each iteration. Subsequently, a simplified algorithm, named LAA, was proposed to reduce the computational complexity and execution time of GAA. In LAA, multiple dominators are elected among one-hop neighbors in each iteration. Moreover, we theoretically proved the correctness and approximation rate of our proposed algorithms. We conducted extensive simulations and the results confirmed the efficiency of our algorithms in prolonging the network lifetime and their effectiveness in constructing an MWmDS.

## References

1. B. Malik, V. Singh, A survey of research in WBAN for biomedical and scientific applications. Health Technol. **3**(3), 227–235 (2013)
2. S.R. Islam, D. Kwak, M.H. Kabir, M. Hossain, K.-S. Kwak, The internet of things for health care: a comprehensive survey. IEEE Access **3**, 678–708 (2015)
3. R.C. Carrano, D. Passos, L.C. Magalhaes, C.V. Albuquerque, Survey and taxonomy of duty cycling mechanisms in wireless sensor networks. IEEE Commun. Surv. Tutorials **16**(1), 181–194 (2014)
4. M. Swaminathan, F.S. Cabrera, J.S. Pujol, U. Muncuk, G. Schirner, K.R. Chowdhury, Multi-path model and sensitivity analysis for galvanic coupled intra-body communication through layered tissue. IEEE Trans. Biomed. Circuits Syst. **10**(2), 339–351 (2016)
5. L. Shi, J. Yuan, S. Yu, M. Li, Mask-ban: movement-aided authenticated secret key extraction utilizing channel characteristics in body area networks. IEEE Internet Things J. **2**(1), 52–62 (2015)

6. R. Zhang, H. Moungla, J. Yu, A. Mehaoua, Medium access for concurrent traffic in wireless body area networks: protocol design and analysis. IEEE Trans. Veh. Technol. **66**(3), 2586–2599 (2017)
7. C. Zhang, Y. Wang, Y. Liang, M. Shu, J. Zhang, L. Ni, Low duty-cycling mac protocol for low data-rate medical wireless body area networks. Sensors **17**(5), 1134 (2017)
8. Q. Shen, W. Zhuang, Energy efficient scheduling for delay constrained communication in wireless body area networks, in *IEEE GLOBECOM* (2012), pp. 262–267
9. H. Li, B. Yang, W. Yu, X. Guan, X. Gong, G. Yu, Joint sleep scheduling and opportunistic transmission in wireless body area networks, in *The 26th IEEE Chinese Control and Decision Conference (CCDC)* (2014), pp. 1886–1891
10. A. Astrin et al., *IEEE Standard for Local and Metropolitan Area Networks - Part 15.6: Wireless Body Area Networks* (2012), pp. 1–271
11. R. Zhang, H. Moungla, A. Mehaoua, A reliable and energy-efficient leader election algorithm for wireless body area networks, in *2015 IEEE International Conference on Communications (ICC)* (IEEE, Piscataway, 2015), pp. 530–535
12. J. Yu, N. Wang, G. Wang, D. Yu, Connected dominating sets in wireless ad hoc and sensor networks–a comprehensive survey. Comput. Commun. **36**(2), 121–134 (2013)
13. Y. Li, Y. Wu, C. Ai, R. Beyah, On the construction of k-connected m-dominating sets in wireless networks. J. Comb. Optim. **23**(1), 118–139 (2012)
14. W. Wang, B. Liu, D. Kim, D. Li, J. Wang, Y. Jiang, A better constant approximation for minimum 3-connected m-dominating set problem in unit disk graph using Tutte decomposition, in *IEEE INFOCOM* (IEEE, Piscataway, 2015), pp. 1796–1804
15. W. Wang, B. Liu, D. Kim, D. Li, J. Wang, W. Gao, A new constant factor approximation to construct highly fault-tolerant connected dominating set in unit disk graph. IEEE/ACM Trans. Netw. (TON) **25**(1), 18–28 (2017)
16. Y. Shi, Z. Zhang, Y. Mo, D.-Z. Du, Approximation algorithm for minimum weight fault-tolerant virtual backbone in unit disk graphs. IEEE/ACM Trans. Netw. (TON) **25**(2), 925–933 (2017)
17. J. Zhou, Z. Zhang, W. Wu, K. Xing, A greedy algorithm for the fault-tolerant connected dominating set in a general graph. J. Comb. Optim. **28**(1), 310–319 (2014)
18. D.Z. Du, K.I. Ko, X. Hu, *Design and Analysis of Approximation Algorithms*, vol. 62 (Springer, Berlin, 2012)
19. E. Reusens, W. Joseph, B. Latré, B. Braem, G. Vermeeren, E. Tanghe, L. Martens, I. Moerman, C. Blondia, Characterization of on-body communication channel and energy efficient topology design for wireless body area networks. IEEE Trans. Inf. Technol. Biomed. **13**(6), 933–945 (2009)
20. R.G. Michael, S.J. David, *Computers and Intractability: A Guide to the Theory of NP-Completeness* (WH Free. Co., San Francisco, 1979), pp. 90–91

# Chapter 6
# Conclusion and Perspective

## 6.1 Book Summary

Recent years have witnessed an unprecedented development of the wireless sensing technology due to its low power and short-range communication pattern. WBSNs have attracted more attention as a new generation of wireless sensing technology, and are used for computer-assisted rehabilitation or continuous health monitoring with real-time updates of medical records through the Internet. As a result, WBSNs are shaping up to be an important part for the Internet of Things (IoT). Although simple to state and intuitively understandable, designing energy-efficient algorithms and protocols require non-trivial efforts to achieve, especially in energy limited WBSNs, due to the particular challenges posed by the WBSNs paradigm.

The above constraints and considerations make energy-efficient algorithms and protocols in this context an emerging research field requiring new tools and methodologies. In this regard, by the present book we hope to make a tiny while systemic step forward in the design and analysis of energy-efficient algorithms and protocols that can scale elegantly, act efficiently in terms of energy, delay, and reliability.

Specifically, this book has been dedicated to addressing the fundamental problem of energy-efficient algorithms and protocols in WBSNs, at both the theoretical modeling and analysis and the practical algorithm design, with Chap. 2 focusing on the clustering-based leader election mechanisms, Chap. 3 proposing duty-cycling MAC protocol for concurrent traffic load, Chap. 4 addressing the multi-channel broadcast problem in asynchronous duty-cycling WBSNs, and Chap. 5 devising a suit of sleep scheduling algorithms for WBSNs to guarantee the network reliability.

More specifically, Chap. 2 first presented a hybrid communication mode such that the burden of the leader and the far node was relived. Correspondingly, a distributed leader election algorithm, EELE, which comprehensively considered both the residual energy and the location of the nodes was developed. The theoretical analysis proved that the overhead of the algorithm was small. Subsequently, the operation of

© Springer Nature Switzerland AG 2020
R. Zhang and J. Yu, *Energy-Efficient Algorithms and Protocols for Wireless Body Sensor Networks*, https://doi.org/10.1007/978-3-030-28580-7_6

the EELE algorithm was introduced in detail. And the simulation results showed that EELE mechanism could reduce the energy consumption, prolong the overall network lifetime, and increase the network throughput effectively.

Moreover, in order to improve the network reliability, we also proceeded to a reliable and energy-efficient leader election scheme in Chap. 2. Specifically, we formulated the reliability model around human body, proposed a reliable and energy-efficient communication strategy, and further analyzed the total energy consumption of a region. Then, a leader election algorithm, REELE, which jointly considered the impact of the reliability, residual energy of a node, and total energy consumption of a region was designed. Extensive simulation results demonstrated the effectiveness and efficiency of REELE in improving the network reliability, besides conserving energy and prolonging network lifetime.

In Chap. 3, we developed a two-phase receiver-initiated asynchronous duty-cycling MAC protocol, called C-MAC, in order to address the delay and energy consumption under concurrent traffic in the medical applications of WBSNs. Specifically, in the first phase, C-MAC employed the IEEE 802.15.6 CSMA/CA mechanism to avoid collisions among control message exchange and sequenced the data packet transmission of different nodes to resolve collisions during the data packet transmission. Moreover, C-MAC enabled nodes to switch to SBM in the second phase, which dramatically reduced the idle listening and overhearing. Subsequently, we explicitly derived the mathematical expressions of delay and energy consumption and further verified their correctness by the numerical analysis and simulation. Furthermore, extensive simulation results verified that the performance of C-MAC in terms of delay and energy consumption outperformed RI-MAC and A-MAC, especially for concurrent traffic.

Chapter 4 first established a theoretical framework on multi-channel broadcast problem in duty-cycling WBSNs and derived the performance bound of any multi-channel broadcast algorithm. Then, with the guidance of theoretical results, we proposed the MCB and improved MCB algorithms to solve the multi-channel broadcast problem guaranteeing the successful broadcast delivery with full diversity regardless of the clock drifts and asymmetric duty cycles. Moreover, we proved the robustness of our MCB algorithms against asymmetrical channel perception within the order-minimal worst-case delay. Finally, the simulation results showed the superiority of our MCB algorithms in reliability and broadcast delay in several typical application scenarios.

Furthermore, in Chap. 5, we first formulated the energy-efficient and reliable sleep scheduling problem in WBSNs via constructing MWmDS and showed its NP-hardness. Then, we introduced a globally optimal approximation algorithm, called GAA, where the node that contributes to the maximum increment of a polymatroid function and residual energy to be the final dominator. Subsequently, an improved local approximation algorithm, named LAA, was presented to reduce the computational complexity and execution time. Moreover, we theoretically proved the correctness and approximation rate of GAA and LAA algorithms. Furthermore, extensive simulation results confirmed the efficiency of our algorithms in prolonging the network lifetime and their effectiveness in constructing an MWmDS.

In what follows, we discuss a number of open questions we judge pertinent to our work and outline several important potential directions for future research.

## 6.2   Open Questions and Future Work

In this section, we develop the discussion on open issues and questions and future work at three levels: the first level focuses on multicast problem, the second one takes the inspiration from the energy harvesting communications, where we plan to tailor efficient algorithms for the problems arising from the new scenarios, and the third one focuses on the generalization of our work in a broader context.

### 6.2.1   Efficient Multicasting Algorithm

In recent years, the energy-efficient multicasting algorithms have been studied in duty-cycling WSNs [1–3], where some approximate scheduling algorithms or greedy algorithms are proposed based on an auxiliary graph to minimize the transmission redundancy, the number of transmissions, and the energy cost during multicasting. However, in healthcare monitoring applications of WBSNs, the sink sometimes also needs to collect specific physiological data from partial sensor nodes instead of all nodes, thus there exists the multicast problem defined as that a control message from the sink should be delivered efficiently to a set of sensor nodes. Therefore, it is necessary to develop the multicasting problems considering the characteristics of WBSNs with the objective to reduce energy consumption and improve time efficiency , especially for duty-cycling and multi-channel WBSNs.

### 6.2.2   Efficient Transmission Strategy with Energy Harvesting

On account of the limited energy capacity, current battery technology does not provide a high enough energy density to develop WBSN nodes with sufficiently long life and acceptable cost. Moreover, the relatively slow rate of progress in battery technology does not promise battery driven sensor nodes in the near future. Furthermore, replacing batteries is simple but not an option in some cases, such as implanted nodes. Energy harvesting has been developed in WSNs [4, 5].

The most promising approach to deal with the energy supply problem for WBSNs is energy harvesting or energy scavenging [6–8]. In this approach, node has an energy harvesting device that collects energy from ambient source such as vibration and motion, light and heat, and radio signals. However, to improve the performance of energy harvesting WBSNs to a level that can be widely adopted, progress needs to be made both in energy harvesting techniques and communication protocols. Harvesting aware communication techniques that take into account and exploit the energy harvesting characteristics are particularly needed to optimize the operations of WBSNs.

To that end, we plan to study the problem of scheduling transmissions in WBSNs with energy harvesting. Specifically, the nodes are assumed to have the ability to choose from a set of available transmission modes, with each scheme consuming a different amount of energy. However, each scheme has a packet error probability that is a decreasing function of the energy used on transmission. Thus we will develop solutions to the following questions: The first one is which transmission mode should be used for a given data packet so as to minimize the probability that the nodes do not have any energy to report future events when they occur while maximizing the likelihood of data reports being correctly transmitted in future work. The second one is on decision making between harvesting energy from radio signal and sending messages at each wake-up slot in duty-cycling WBSNs.

## 6.2.3  Extension to Cloud Computing

In this book, we mainly focused on the energy-efficient algorithms and protocols design and analysis in WBSNs. In WBSNs, both the sensing data and the feedback from a doctor should be timely processed. Moreover, the increasing demands from customers and patients consume more network resources, i.e., storage, computation, and communication power, but it is difficult to achieve these goals only relying on the traditional WBSNs. Therefore, the cloud computing is introduced to assist WBSNs to store and process the sensing data in a real-time fashion [9, 10]. Taking the advantage of the cloud server to store the large volume of sensing data and process them for doctor's diagnosis, cloud assisted WBSNs become more robust and provide the desirable services for patients and users. However, when a large number of users located at the same place upload their data at the same time, the connection between WBSNs and cloud servers might be intermittent. The available bandwidths from WBSNs to cloud servers for each individual user are also limited so that the network performance is considerably degraded. Therefore, the communication between WBSNs and cloud servers is the bottleneck with the perspective of efficiency and reliability. We plan to design a suitable scheme to handle the challenges.

## References

1. Q. Chen, S. Cheng, H. Gao, J. Li, Z. Cai, Energy-efficient algorithm for multicasting in duty-cycled sensor networks. Sensors **15**(12), 31224–31243 (2015)
2. Q. Chen, H. Gao, S. Cheng, Z. Cai, Approximate scheduling and constructing algorithms for minimum-energy multicasting in duty-cycled sensor networks, in *2015 International Conference on Identification, Information, and Knowledge in the Internet of Things (IIKI)* (IEEE, Piscataway, 2015), pp. 163–168

3. K. Verma, Multicast routing protocols for wireless sensor networks: a comparative study. Int. J. Comput. Sci. **2015**(1) (2015)
4. F.K. Shaikh, S. Zeadally, Energy harvesting in wireless sensor networks: a comprehensive review. Renew. Sust. Energy Rev. **55**, 1041–1054 (2016)
5. X. Lu, P. Wang, D. Niyato, D.I. Kim, Z. Han, Wireless networks with RF energy harvesting: a contemporary survey. IEEE Commun. Surv. Tutorials **17**(2), 757–789 (2015)
6. S. Yousaf, N. Javaid, U. Qasim, N. Alrajeh, Z.A. Khan, M. Ahmed, Towards reliable and energy-efficient incremental cooperative communication for wireless body area networks. Sensors **16**(3), 284 (2016)
7. X. Xu, L. Shu, M. Guizani, M. Liu, J. Lu, A survey on energy harvesting and integrated data sharing in wireless body area networks. Int. J. Distrib. Sens. Netw. **2015**, 5 (2015)
8. S. Liu, K. Wang, J. Guo, Y. Wang, X. Qi, Review on mac protocols in energy harvesting wireless body area networks, in *2015 International Conference on Identification, Information, and Knowledge in the Internet of Things (IIKI)* (IEEE, Piscataway, 2015), pp. 303–304
9. J. Zhou, Z. Cao, X. Dong, N. Xiong, A.V. Vasilakos, 4s: a secure and privacy-preserving key management scheme for cloud-assisted wireless body area network in m-healthcare social networks. Inf. Sci. **314**, 255–276 (2015)
10. S. Moulik, S. Misra, A. Gaurav, Cost-effective mapping between wireless body area networks and cloud service providers based on multi-stage bargaining. IEEE Trans. Mobile Comput. **16**(6), 1573–1586 (2016)

# Index

**A**

Actuators, 1, 40
Ad hoc sensor networks, 14
A-MAC, 42, 124
 delay analysis, 65–67
 energy consumption, 67–69
Antenna design, 7
Asynchronous duty-cycling MAC protocols,
  41
 comparison, 43, 44
 concurrent traffic load (*see* C-MAC
   protocol)
 receiver-initiated protocols, 42–43
 sender-initiated protocols, 42
Asynchronous duty-cycling WBSNs, 123


**B**

BD, *see* Broadcast delay
BD-FD, *see* Broadcast delay with full diversity
Bit error rate (BER), 4
Bluetooth low energy (BLE), 4–5
Bluetooth technology, 4–5
B-MAC, 42
Broadcast delay (BD), 80, 124
 multi-channel case, 88
  asymmetrical channel perceptions,
   98–99
  average BD-FD, 95, 96
  average first BD, 96, 97
  BD-FD *vs.* number of channels, 96, 98
  simulation results, 96
  worst-case BD-FD, 95
  worst-case first BD, 96, 97

 single-channel case, 86
  average BD, 93, 94
  simulation results, 93, 95
  worst-case BD, 93, 94
Broadcast delay with full diversity (BD-FD),
  80
 average BD-FD, 95, 96
 *vs.* number of channels, 96, 98
 worst-case BD-FD, 95
Broadcast diversity, 79–81, 88


**C**

Channel access, 4–6
Channel hopping schedule, 78–79
Chinese remainder theorem (CRT), 83–84, 86,
  88, 90
Clock drifts, 83–86, 88, 93
 definition, 79
 duty cycle and, 80, 124
 offset, 88
Cloud computing, 126
Cluster-based topology, 16
Cluster head selection, 12, 13
 broadcasting advertisement
   message, 13
 clustering protocols, 16
 HEED approach, 14
 LEACH protocol, 13–14
 M-EECP, 14
 S-EECP, 14
Clustering-based leader election mechanisms,
  123
Cluster members, 13

C-MAC protocol
    collision, 40, 41
    control message exchange phase, 46, 47
    data packet transmission, 124
    data packet transmission phase, 46, 47
    delay ($T_d$) analysis, 124
        accuracy evaluation, 60–61
        for arbitrary node, 49
        average delay with different duty cycles,
            66, 67
        average delay with different traffic
            loads, 65, 66
        components, 49
        modeling of $T_1$, 51–52
        modeling of $T_o$ and $T_o$, 59–60
        modeling of $T_w$, 53–59
        RI-MAC vs. A-MAC, 65–67
        symbols used, 49–51
    energy consumption, 124
        accuracy evaluation, 64
        modeling of, 62–64
        RI-MAC vs. A-MAC, 67–69
    idle listening, 40, 41
    IEEE 802.15.6 CSMA/CA mechanism, 40,
        45–46, 124
    operation of, 46
    ordering-based communication algorithm,
        41, 47–49
    overhearing, 40, 41
    random delay, 41
    simulation settings, 65
    standby mode, 41
Coexistence, 3
Cognitive radio ad hoc networks, 76–77
Communication range, 3
Computational complexity, 111, 112, 114–115,
    124
Connected dominating set (CDS), 104
Control message exchange phase, 46, 47, 124
CRT, see Chinese remainder theorem


D
Data packet transmission phase, 46–48
Data rate, 3–6, 40, 42, 60
Distance-aware hybrid communication
    approach, 12, 15
Distributed leader election algorithm, 12, 15,
    17, 37, 123
Dominating set (DS), 102
    cardinality of, 115, 118, 119
    dominatees, 105, 111
    dominators, 105, 111, 112
    execution rounds, 118, 119

$m$-fold, 104–105, 108, 113, 114
    of sensor nodes, 106, 107
Domination capability, 112, 114, 117
DS, see Dominating set
Duty cycle
    arbitrary, 74
    asymmetric, 74, 78, 93, 124
    average delay with, 65, 66
    definition, 79
    granularity, 75, 85–86, 89, 95
    heterogeneous, 74, 75
    node's, 83
    operation mode, 73
    reciprocals of, 82, 84, 93, 95, 96
    WiseMAC, 42
Duty cycled multi-hop wireless networks,
    76
Duty-cycling MAC protocols
    active state, 44
    asynchronous duty-cycling MAC protocols,
        41
        comparison, 43, 44
        concurrent traffic load (see C-MAC
            protocol)
        receiver-initiated protocols, 42–43
        sender-initiated protocols, 42
    for concurrent traffic load, 123
    sleep state, 44
    standby state, 44
    state transition relationship, 44, 45
    synchronous duty-cycling MAC protocols,
        40, 41
Duty-cycling WBSNs, 102
    asynchronous, 123
    MAC protocols (see Duty-cycling MAC
        protocols)
    MCB algorithms (see Multi-channel
        broadcast algorithms)


E
EELE, see Energy-efficient leader election
    mechanism
Energy efficiency
    of broadcasting, 76
    of clustering protocol, 13, 15
    definition, 36
    EELE (see Energy-efficient leader election
        mechanism)
    of LEACH-A, 36
    MAC protocol, 6–7, 40
    network layer, 7
    REELE (see Reliable and energy-efficient
        leader election algorithm)

Energy-efficient cooperative relay selection
        scheme, 14
Energy-efficient leader election (EELE)
        mechanism, 12, 123–124
    distance-aware hybrid communication
        approach, 15
    distributed leader election algorithm, 15
    energy consumption-based hybrid
        communication strategy, 17–18
    initial phase, 21
    leader election algorithm, 18–20
    operation
        flowchart, 22
        time line, 20, 21
    performance evaluation, LEACH-A vs.
        HEED-A
        $\alpha$ on network lifetime, 24
        alive nodes over time, 24, 26
        average residual energy over time, 25,
            26
        dead nodes and alive nodes, 24, 25
        energy characteristics, 22
        network energy efficiency over time,
            25, 27
        network lifetime, 22
        residual energy, 23–24
        sensor location, 23
        simulation parameters, 23, 24
        throughput, 22
        throughput over different initial energy,
            27, 28
    scheduling phase, 21
    set-up phase, 21
    steady-state phase, 21
Energy harvesting, 7, 125–126
Enhancement of low energy adaptive clustering
        hierarchy (e-LEACH), 13
European Telecommunication Standard
        Institute (ETSI), 6

**F**
Fault-tolerant CDS, 104

**G**
GAA, see Global approximation algorithm
G-ACK, see Group-ACK
Global approximation algorithm (GAA), 103,
        108, 109, 124
    analysis, 110–111
    design, 109–110

DS cardinality and execution rounds,
        119–120
    network lifetime, 117–119
Greedy algorithm, 105, 111, 125
Group-ACK (G-ACK), 47, 59, 63, 69

**H**
HEED-Analogous (HEED-A), 17
    vs. EELE and LEACH-A, 24–27
    vs. REELE and LEACH-A, 33–37
HEED approach, see Hybrid energy-efficient
        distributed cluster approach
Hybrid communication mode, 17, 18, 123
Hybrid energy-efficient distributed cluster
        (HEED) approach, 12, 14, 17

**I**
IEEE 802.15.6 CSMA/CA mechanism, 40,
        45–47, 51, 124
IEEE 802.15.4 standard, 5
IEEE 802.15.6 standard, 5–6
Immediate-ACK (I-ACK), 47
Improved MCB
    improved algorithm, 89–90
    vs. MCB vs. Random reliability, 92–99
    robustness against asymmetrical channel
        perception, 90–92
Interference, 3–5, 74
Internet of Things (IoT), 123

**K**
km-CDS, 104

**L**
LAA, see Local approximation algorithm
Langford Paring and Skolem sequence,
        77
Latency, 3
    BLE, 4
    IEEE 802.15.4, 5
    minimum latency broadcast schedule, 76
    in packet delivery, 43
    sensor nodes, 39
LEACH-Analogous (LEACH-A), 17
    vs. EELE and HEED-A, 24–28
    vs. REELE and HEED-A, 34–37
LEACH protocol, see Low energy adaptive
        cluster hierarchy protocol

Leader election algorithm
    distributed, 13, 15, 17, 37, 123
    EELE, 18–20
    REELE, 32–33, 124
Line-of-signal (LOS) channel, 17
Local approximation algorithm (LAA), 103,
        108, 124
    analysis, 113–115
    computational complexity, 111
    design, 111–113
    domination capability, 117
    DS cardinality and execution rounds,
        119–120
    network lifetime, 117–119
Low energy adaptive cluster hierarchy
        (LEACH) protocol, 13–14, 17
Low power listening (LPL) mechanism, 42
Lyapunov optimization, 103


**M**
MAC layer design, 6–7
MAC protocols
    duty-cycling (*see* Duty-cycling MAC
        protocols)
    MAC layer design, 6–7
MCB algorithms, *see* Multi-channel broadcast
        algorithms
$m$-fold CDS, 104
Minimum weighted $m$-fold dominating set
        (MWmDS) problem, 102
    GAA (*see* Global approximation algorithm)
    LAA (*see* Local approximation algorithm)
    in NP-hardness, 103, 108, 124
Multicasting algorithm, 125
Multi-channel broadcast (MCB) algorithms
    asymmetrical channel perception, 124
    channel hopping sequence, 77
    cognitive radio ad hoc networks, 76–77
    delay bound, 81–82
    duty-cycling broadcast problem, 76
    heterogeneous duty cycles, 75
    improved MCB
        improved algorithm, 89–90
        robustness against asymmetrical
            channel perception, 90–92
        MCB *vs.* improved MCB *vs.* random
            reliability, 92–93
    minimum latency broadcast schedule, 76
    multi-channel case
        broadcast delay, 88, 95–99
        motivation and algorithm design, 86–88
    multi-channel communication pattern, 76
    optimal problem, 80–81

    performance metrics, 80
    rendezvous channel, 77
    requirements, 74
    simplicial-complex-based broadcast
        algorithm, 77
    single-channel case
        algorithm design, 84–85
        broadcast delay, 86, 93–95
        Chinese remainder theorem, 83–84
        duty cycle granularity, 85–86
    single-channel environment, 76
    sink and sensor nodes, 73–75
    system model, 78–79
    wake-up schedules, 76, 77
Multi-hop energy-efficient clustering protocol
        (M-EECP), 14
MWmDS problem, *see* Minimum weighted
        $m$-fold dominating set problem


**N**
Network density, 3
Network layer design, 7
Node identification number (NID), 16, 19, 21,
        31
Non-cluster head nodes, 13, 14
Non-line-of-signal (NLOS) channel, 17


**O**
O-ACK, *see* Organized-ACK
Ordering-based communication algorithm, 41,
        47–49
Order-minimal worst-case delay, 75, 124
Organized-ACK (O-ACK), 47–49, 59, 63
Outage probability, 12, 15, 30


**P**
Packet error rate probability, 12, 15
Packet loss probability, 4
Path loss, 12, 15, 28–29, 104, 107
    coefficient, 17, 106
    and shadowing effects, 102
    total path loss, 29
Personal digital assistant (PDA), 1, 11
PHY layer design, 6
Polymatroid function, 103, 105, 108–111, 124
PW-MAC, 43


**R**
Realistic nonlinear energy consumption model,
    14
Receiver-centric MAC (RC-MAC) protocol, 43

Receiver-initiated protocols (RI-MAC), 42–43, 124
  delay analysis, 65–67
  energy consumption, 67–69
REELE, see Reliable and energy-efficient leader election algorithm
Region identification number (RID), 16, 19–21, 32
Reliability, 3–4, 13, 27, 104, 110, 124
  MCB vs. improved MCB vs. Random, 92–93
  QoS and, 8
  REELE (see Reliable and energy-efficient leader election algorithm)
Reliable and energy-efficient leader election (REELE) algorithm, 12, 27
  effectiveness and efficiency, 124
  leader election algorithm, 124
  performance evaluation, LEACH-A vs. HEED-A
    average residual energy over time, 34, 35
    energy consumption of leader, 36, 37
    energy efficiency over time, 34–36
    network lifetime over initial energy, 34
    reliability of each node, 37
  reliability model, 28–29
  reliable and energy-efficient communication strategy, 30
  reliable leader election algorithm, 31–33
  total energy consumption model, 30–31
Reliable leader election algorithm, 32–33
RI-MAC, see Receiver-initiated protocols

S
SBM, see Standby mode
Scalability, 4, 5, 13, 16
Simplicial-complex-based broadcast algorithm, 77
Single-hop energy-efficient clustering protocol (S-EECP), 14
Sleep scheduling algorithms
  connected dominating set, 104
  dominating set, 102
  greedy algorithm, 105
  Lyapunov optimization theory, 103
  m-fold dominating set, 104–105
  minimum submodular cover problem, 105
  MWmDS problem
    GAA (see Global approximation algorithm)

LAA (see Local approximation algorithm)
  in NP-hardness, 103, 108, 124
  and opportunistic transmission policy, 103
  performance evaluation
    DS cardinality, 115
    execution rounds, 116
    network lifetime, 115
    simulation parameters, 115
    simulation results, 116–120
  polymatroid function, 105
  problem formulation, 107–108
  system model, 106, 107
  tuning parameter, 103
  two-hop communication, 104
  two-step scheduling algorithm, 103
SmartBAN, 6
Standby mode (SBM), 41, 44, 47, 60, 63, 68, 124
Synchronous duty-cycling MAC protocols, 40, 41

T
TAD-MAC protocol, see Traffic-aware dynamic MAC protocol
TID, see Type identification number
Total energy consumption model, 13, 22, 30–31, 34, 36, 62, 124
Traffic-aware dynamic MAC (TAD-MAC) protocol, 43
Transmission strategy, 125–126
Two-hop communication, 104
Two-hop cooperative communication, 12, 15
Two-phase receiver-initiated duty-cycling protocol, 103, 124
Two-step scheduling algorithm, 103
Type identification number (TID), 16, 19–21

W
WBSNs, see Wireless body sensor networks
Wireless body sensor networks (WBSNs)
  actuators, 1
  broadcast algorithm
    asynchronous local clocks, 74
    clock synchronization, 74
    duty cycle operation mode, 73
    multi-channel broadcast problem, 74
    multi-channel communication pattern (see Multi-channel broadcast algorithms)

Wireless body sensor networks (WBSNs)
        (*cont.*)
    cloud computing, 126
    design requirement, 3–4
    duty-cycling
        asynchronous, 123
        MAC protocols (*see* Duty-cycling MAC
            protocols)
        MCB algorithms (*see* Multi-channel
            broadcast algorithms)
    energy conservation
        cluster head selection (*see* Cluster head
            selection)
        clustering methodology, 12
        clustering protocols, 15
        cluster members, 13
        EELE (*see* Energy-efficient leader
            election mechanism)
        energy-efficient cooperative relay
            selection scheme, 15
        HEED, 12
        network model, 16–17
        packet error rate *vs.* transmitted power,
            12, 15
        REELE (*see* Reliable and energy-
            efficient leader election algorithm)
        two-hop cooperative communication,
            12
    energy consumption and latency, 39
    energy-efficient algorithms and protocols,
        123
    health care monitoring, 39
    healthcare monitoring applications, 125
    IoT, 123
    limited energy resource, 101–102
    low-power sensor nodes, 101
    medical and non-medical applications

    healthcare, 1–2
    military and defense, 2
    sport and entertainment, 2
multicasting algorithm, 125
multi-channel, 125
open issues and challenges
    antenna design, 7
    energy supply, 7
    MAC layer design, 6–7
    network layer design, 7
    PHY layer design, 6
    QoS and reliability, 8
    security and privacy, 8
personal digital assistant, 1
sensors, 1
sink, 11, 101
sleep scheduling algorithms (*see* Sleep
        scheduling algorithms)
transmission strategy with energy
        harvesting, 125–126
unstable wireless channel, 102
wireless technologies
    Bluetooth, 4–5
    IEEE 802.15.4, 5
    IEEE 802.15.6, 5–6
    SmartBAN, 6
    ZigBee, 5
Wireless personal area networks (WPAN), 5
WiseMAC, 42

**X**
X-MAC, 42

**Z**
ZigBee, 5

Printed in the United States
By Bookmasters